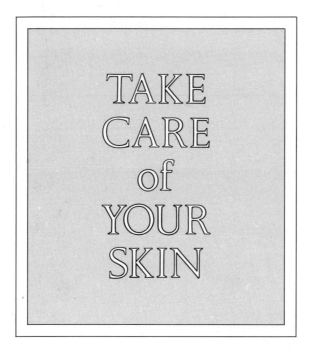

TAKE
CARE
of
YOUR
SKIN

Also by Elaine Brumberg
Save Your Money, Save Your Face

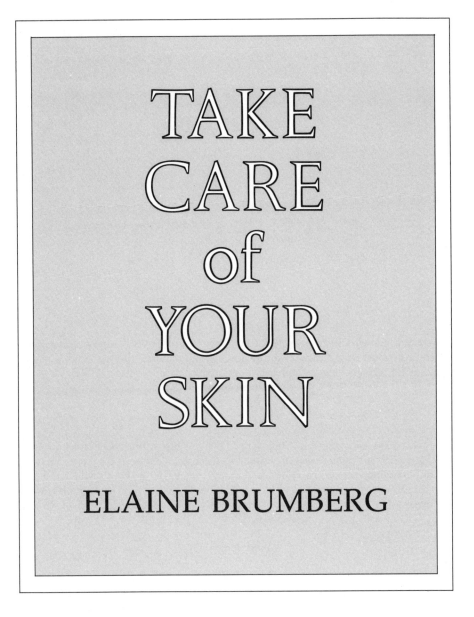

TAKE CARE of YOUR SKIN

ELAINE BRUMBERG

1817

HARPER & ROW, PUBLISHERS, New York
Grand Rapids, Philadelphia, St. Louis, San Francisco
London, Singapore, Sydney, Tokyo

Grateful acknowledgment is made for permission to reprint in Chapter 10 the Skin Cancer Foundation's guidelines for identifying and reducing the risk of melanoma and list of recommended sunscreens. Reprinted by permission of the Skin Cancer Foundation.

FIRST EDITION

Designed by Mary Beth Kilkelly/Levavi & Levavi

Library of Congress Cataloging-in-Publication Data

Brumberg, Elaine.
    Take care of your skin / Elaine Brumberg. — 1st ed.
       p.   cm.
    Includes index.
    ISBN 0-06-015793-3 :
    1. Skin—Care and hygiene. 2. Cosmetics. 3. Consumer education. I. Title.
RL87.B78   1989
646.7'26—dc19
                                     88-45888

89 90 91 92 93 CC/RRD 10 9 8 7 6 5 4 3 2 1

This book is dedicated to my family, particularly my best friend, lover, and husband, Norman; my children, Amy, Bruce, Harriet, and Scott; and my beautiful granddaughter, Ilyse Beth Kramer.

CONTENTS

FOUR: DESIGNING YOUR OWN SKIN CARE
PROGRAM: KNOWING WHAT TO BUY AND
HOW TO USE IT

FOREWORD

In our quest for beauty and perpetual youth, women are often misled into believing that there are solutions, or that there actually is a single solution, to both. We use lotions and potions, camouflage makeups and removers, in an attempt to fix or to cover existing defects in our skin. Often the means of preventing the defect before it appears is completely ignored.

In my dermatology practice, the most common complaints that my female patients have about their skin relate to either acne or aging skin. There are numerous presentations to both conditions and each has a different solution. For instance, the fourteen-year-old girl with adolescent acne requires a unique approach, as does the twenty-eight-year-old woman and the forty-year-old. One has skin that is oily yet sensitive, another may have hormonally active skin, and the next has skin which is dry but still acne-prone. Each of these patients might be using ten treatment products, and chances are the products are at odds with the problem they were bought to correct.

Aging skin is a special problem that generates much emotional turmoil in many women, even those in their mid- to late twenties. Much of this could have been avoided had the sun not played such a prominent role in most of our youth. Days at the beach with baby oil and reflectors, college vacations spent basking in the Florida sun, and Caribbean vacations have been the norm for many of us. Fortunately, I see a trend away from this foolish behavior in many of my female patients, who are unhappy with the brown spots (solar keratoses, in medical terms) on their faces, chests, and hands, the scaly patches (also solar keratoses) on their faces, and fine wrinkles. We are now angry with ourselves for having allowed this to happen to us (and how slowly this sun damage sneaks up on us!) and are determined to remedy it as quickly as possible.

Of course, if there really were one product that could reverse all signs of aging, the world would embrace it at once. Retin-A may be the closest thing to a "miracle solution" that has been seen in this century. We are still not sure what impact Retin-A will have on this whole issue. However, it has been used for several decades in the treatment of acne and appears to have no negative effects. The biggest problems I see with Retin-A are that it is sometimes used in women with such advanced skin aging that it would be impossible to see much benefit and that it is sometimes prescribed by physicians who have little or no experience in using it. This can result in severe irritant reactions, severe sunburn, and in general misery for the unfortunate user. It is not wise to borrow one's friend's tube of Retin-A, either! The final answer is not in on this drug, but it does seem to hold much promise.

But aside from this actual treatment for aging (and acne, for that matter), how are women to approach their own skin care when confronted with so much information through advertising and salesmanship? Elaine Brumberg has long been involved in trying to turn us from disheartened and uneducated consumers into satisfied and savvy ones. She gives the reader a framework for understanding the skin's structure and function so that our approach is an intelligent one. Once we understand our skin type and its unique reactions, women are in a better position to judge which products might best serve to enhance it. The messages that Ms. Brumberg delivers include avoidance of sun as an important ingredient in skin care, as well as recognition of the types of products that will interact most favorably with one's skin. However, often these two elements still do not correct the problems, and the help of a dermatologist should be sought.

I have a double perspective, as both a dermatologist and a skin care consumer. It is imperative that dermatologists keep themselves abreast of what's out there, what their patients are using, and what benefits there are to women taking charge of their own treatment regimens. It is not acceptable to be told by a dermatologist in a huff that soap and water are fine, just use any moisturizer, and forget all masks and toners. Many are actually helpful for the physical or mental well-being of our patients and we cannot be so quick to dismiss them.

Armed with sturdy background information and a good understanding of their own skin, women, their dermatologists, and skin care companies can and should become fast friends.

—Ellen C. Gendler, M.D.

ACKNOWLEDGMENTS

The most important person I would like to thank is Julia Coopersmith. Her research, organization, talent, and hard work made all of this possible. I also want to give a very special thank you to the following: my editors at Harper & Row, Carol Cohen and Helen Moore, for their support and guidance; Joseph Montebello, the creative director at Harper & Row, for the elegant book design; my son Bruce Brumberg, Esq., for his thorough research; and my son-in-law, Robert Kramer, Esq., for all his wonderful legal advice. I am particularly grateful to Dr. Roger Schnaare for his patience and valuable information.

Many other individuals and organizations have contributed invaluable help: Patricia Mullings, Lou Rothman, Carol Firsching, and Theresa Rooney from Cosmetic City, Elkins Park, Pennsylvania; Joyce Ayoub from the Skin Cancer Foundation, New York City; and Jack Shalita, Fred Cohen, and Jack Meehan from the Bethayres Pharmacy, Huntingdon Valley, Pennsylvania.

I would like to acknowledge and thank Dr. Heinz J. Eirmann, director of the FDA's Cosmetic Division, for his kindness and cooperation in sharing so much information and Gary Grove, Ph.D., vice president of research and development of KGL's Skin Study Center, for so generously contributing his time and information.

There is no way to appropriately thank the physicians who so generously gave of their time and knowledge: Dr. Albert Kligman, Dr. Paul Gross, Dr. Myron Rosenfeld, Dr. James Slavin, Dr. Barrett Noone, and Dr. Magdi S. Kodsi.

I would like to also thank treasured friends and extraordinary women Linda Schwartz, Frieda Cotler, Paula Magan, Dora Schwartz, Ruth Mantin, Beth D'Addano, Stephanie Block Sherman, Carol Strange, Joanne Stoloff, Ruth Samuels, Sylvia Mott, Judy Podwil, Carolyn Lusch, Pat Gavaghan, Roz Marion, Betty Lennon, and Alice Zemble.

A sincere and profound thanks to my hairdresser Joseph Langsdorf, makeup artist Peter Brown, and photographer John Gregory.

And last but not least I would like to acknowledge the Clairton High School Class of 1958.

ONE

Skin Care Products: Why We Buy Them/ How They Sell Them

1

What Kind of Skin Care Consumer Are You?

Yes, absolutely, I try to take care of my skin. I use Jergens on my whole body after I shower, and every night I put cream on my face. I have my whole life . . . I use either Oil of Olay or Nivea or sometimes just plain Vaseline. I guess you could say I am totally hooked on face cream.

—MARGERY S., SIXTY-SIX-YEAR-OLD RETIRED LIBRARIAN

The American consumer spends more than two and one-half billion dollars annually on products such as moisturizers, cleansers, and anti-aging creams. Skin care products took their biggest leap forward in the early 1980s, when sales jumped more than 26 percent, and skin care is still the fastest growing segment of the cosmetics industry.

In my work, I talk to a lot of women about their skin care needs, and I have not yet met a single woman who did not use some form of skin care product. Young women, old women, middle-aged women, without exception, find cleansers and moisturizers as much a part of their daily routines as toothbrushes.

As I expected, the younger woman was thinking about oil control, the older woman was worried about dry skin, and the middle-aged woman was deciding whether or not she should sample products with anti-aging claims. I did, however, have several misconceptions about the skin care consumer. I had assumed that the women who spent a lot on makeup preparations would be the same ones who indulged in expensive face creams, and vice versa, but my research did not indicate that this was necessarily the case. I met many women who wore little if any makeup and then surprised me by saying that they thought so-called anti-aging moisturizing preparations were a necessity.

By and large, though, all of the women I met were confused about what skin care products they should use. Bombarded by advertisements and exotic packaging, the average consumer is both curious and skeptical about the claims for newer products. I found that most women act out this curiosity and skepticism in the following way: On the one hand, they tend to cling to old skin care rituals as well as tried and true product choices. On the other, they make occasional forays into department stores and drug outlets, where they buy one or more of the newer lotions and potions—usually in response to a particular advertisement.

My friend Mary is a good example of a woman who indulges in this kind of behavior:

> I've been doing the same thing for years. I wash my face with soap and water in the shower every morning. This makes it feel very dry, so then I use a lot of moisturizer—Oil of Olay, to be specific. When I go to bed I use Nivea Oil. Basically, that's all I do *regularly.* However, about once or twice a year, usually when I'm worried about finding and keeping love in my life, I read a magazine article, or see an advertisement that makes me want to go out and hit the stores. This is a very expensive diversion, but I bought CHR Pro-Collagen this way and Glycel night cream and Adrien Arpel Hydro-Cellular Serum and, recently, Avon's Line Controlling lotion from an Avon representative. I liked the Glycel night cream, but I didn't think it was worth $70. The Collagen Booster I didn't understand probably because it doesn't look like cream.
>
> I'm not sure what to do with it. The Adrien Arpel felt good, but I didn't buy it again because I didn't want to spend the money. The Pro-Collagen might be a great product, but, again, it didn't look like anything I was accustomed to, and I didn't really give it a chance. I guess I expected to see something dramatically different on my face immediately. I didn't, so I gave up.

The Mistakes We Make and How to Avoid Them

Let's face it, when dealing with cosmetics companies, inflated advertising claims seem to come with the territory. It appears as though nearly every marketeer has come up with a product that was "designed" to "help" wipe out the "effects of aging" by "smoothing away" and/or "preventing" wrinkling. These ads are carefully designed to influence you, the skin care consumer.

Since I definitely want to belong to the smooth-faced generation, I guess if it wasn't for the money involved I would want to buy and try everything. But I can't afford to do that, and I don't know many women who can. Skin care products are simply too expensive for us to risk many mistakes.

Nonetheless, I have found that the typical consumer does make mistakes primarily because she wants to believe in miracles. She tends to go off to buy the newest advertised skin care products without even a rudimentary understanding of what the ads are selling, what the products are promising, or what she wants. When this happens, the woman more often than not becomes discouraged because the product doesn't seem to be doing what she hoped for, and she goes back to her old stand-by, which often is a less expensive product that has served her in good stead for many years. I call this "hit and miss" shopping. The only problem with this approach is that a woman's skin care needs change not only as she ages, but also with the seasons, and sometimes she is not taking this into consideration.

In my opinion, looking for miraculous results is one of the primary reasons for hit and miss cosmetics consumerism. Buying skin care products should be a totally practical matter. Here are some of the kinds of things you should ask yourself before heading for the store:

A Skin Care Quiz

1. Skin type changes as we age. Are you *absolutely* certain about your skin type or are you assuming that it is the same as it was five or ten years ago?
2. Most, if not all, skin care products are designed with specific skin types in mind. Do you know how to determine which products are appropriate for you?

3. Skin care advertisements toss around a lot of fancy words. Do you know the difference between an emollient and a humectant? How about dermis and epidermis?

4. Sunscreens are given numbers to indicate their SPF (Sun Protection Factor). Do you know which number is right for you?

5. Sunscreens have traditionally protected against ultraviolet B, but new evidence indicates that ultraviolet A is also implicated in skin damage. Do you know how, and are you using a product that screens out both ultraviolet A and B?

6. Many scientific experts believe that something called the free radical is implicated in the aging process. Do you know what a free radical is? Do you know which skin care ingredients help protect against the free radicals?

7. Cell turnover is a phrase that is used in many skin care ads. Do you know what it means, and how much or how little skin care products affect it?

8. Women in their twenties with normal skin often precipitate their own skin problems by purchasing products designed for mature dry skin. If you have normal skin, do you know which ingredients are too "rich" for your skin type?

9. Cleansing products, including scrubs and masks, can sometimes cause more harm than good. Do you know why?

10. The "look" of aging skin often appears because skin cells of a mature woman do not retain as much moisture. Do you know which ingredients are more effective in binding water to your skin and help give the skin a more youthful appearance?

11. Advertisements and labels for expensive anti-aging products often refer to different types of ingredients. Do you know, for example, anything about the following: hyaluronic acid, mucopolysaccharide, NMF, retinyl palmitate, ascorbic acid?

12. When you go to buy cosmetics, the salesperson often suggests that you buy several products from the same line. Is it preferable to stick to one skin care program or can you mix and match?

13. Many skin care consumers are brand loyal. If this is the case with you, do you know why you have these feelings?

14. Certain masks and cleansing-type products achieve good results. However, the same results can be achieved for pennies using ordinary household ingredients. Do you really believe this, and do you know what to do?

15. Most of the women I talked to told me that money was a big factor in how they purchased skin care products. Do you have a skin care budget as well as an effective plan to get the best value for your cosmetic dollar?

Learning the answers to these questions—and others—is the best way I can think of to protect yourself from advertising hype and make you a smart skin care consumer.

Is There Any Truth in the Hype?

One of the questions I am asked all the time is whether I think it's all hype, and the typical question put to me is, "When it comes to skin care products, is there any truth in advertising?" Do any of these products have any real value?

The skin care consumer—and that means you and me—is exposed to a great a deal of hype. Buying into this hype means you run the risk of wasting money, buying the wrong skin care products, or possibly creating dermatological problems.

However, I also believe that many skin care products improve a woman's appearance, but there is so much overselling and promotional hype that it is difficult for the average woman to find the products that work for her.

From where I sit, there are strong pros and strong cons. When I'm asked my opinion on the skin care industry, I often think of two different stories that I would like to share with you:

Skin Care Products—A Good Story: Or, How $12.50 Worth of Moisturizer Helped Restore the Confidence of an Eighty-Six-Year-Old Woman My mother-in-law, a wonderful woman, now in her eighties, lives in Florida. About three and a half years ago, she called me on the phone and asked me whether or not I would recommend that she start using an anti-aging cream. Did I think, she inquired, it would make her skin look younger and more radiant.

She assured me that she was no stranger to skin care; she had always used cold cream, Pond's to be exact, after showering. But she had never done anything fancy, and, basically, she was an old-fashioned soap-and-water lady. She said she wanted to stay that way and didn't want to try anything complicated, but she had been looking at magazine ads, and the advertising copy was promising. She was tired of always having dry skin and she wondered if maybe an anti-aging moisturizing cream might help.

Well, the next time she came to visit, I bought her a collagen-based moisturizer from a private label company in my area, and she immediately began applying it in the morning and in the evening.

A couple of months went by before she phoned to say that she had a new and very attentive boyfriend. My husband and I think that her suitor was attracted to her personality and joie de vivre, but she claims that the moisturizer helped. She said she definitely felt it improved her overall appearance. She said her skin looked better, she looked better, and she absolutely felt better because of it.

I cannot deny that $12.50 worth of moisturizer improved my mother-in-law's self confidence. It definitely made her skin feel softer and it improved moisture retention. Whether or not it reduced wrinkling is debatable, but she perceives her skin as being less wrinkled, and I am not going to argue with her. My mother-in-law needs a new supply of moisturizer every two and a half months, therefore it costs her about $60 a year to get enough results to make her happy. This is a very modest sum to spend.

Whenever women ask me about the benefits of skin care products, I think of my mother-in-law. Hers was a very happy experience, and her collagen-based moisturizer worked for her.

But there is another story that I remember. This is another woman's experience, and it is a good example of how a cosmetic sales pitch can affect a woman who is feeling personally vulnerable.

Skin Care Products—A Nightmare: Or, How a $25 Facial and $134 Worth of Face Creams Turned a Twenty-Six-Year-Old Ivory Girl into a Skin Care Casualty   Debbie is a woman I met while I was traveling. Distressed about a bad experience with skin care products, she was anxious to talk to me about it. About a year ago, she spotted a department store ad that appealed to her. A major cosmetics company was making the following offer: For under $25 an expert would do a minifacial and a cosmetic makeover. The customer would also receive a small makeup bag and samples of four of the company's skin care products.

Debbie was trying to make a career change, and when she went on interviews, she wanted to look her best. She felt an improved appearance would improve her confidence. Twenty-five dollars for a facial seemed like a small price to pay for more confidence.

Debbie had limited experience with skin care products. She still used Noxzema exactly as she had when she was a teenager. She used light makeup and washed her face with soap. That was it. As a teenager, she had a tendency toward mild acne breakouts—nothing serious—but she made a point of washing her face several times a day because oil would collect in the pores around her nose and chin and she wanted to avoid blackheads.

On the day of the facial, when she arrived at the store, an attractive young woman ushered her onto a stool, covered her in plastic, and began smearing white stuff on her face. No one asked her skin type, and no one seemed to act as though it made any difference.

The cosmetics expert used tissue to wipe off the cream, and then put another creamy substance on her face. She then started in with a brush that massaged the skin with the cream, which Debbie thinks was a scrub cleanser. Then that was rubbed off with a damp cotton ball, and an astringent was used. The expert told Debbie that her skin was dehydrated and applied a mask that she said would help. She also pointed out that Debbie was forming fine lines around her eyes and would need an eye cream. She applied a very greasy substance around Debbie's eyes. There were several other women sitting on stools. They were also receiving facials, and Debbie couldn't help but notice that all of their faces looked red and irritated, but when Debbie asked the expert about it, she was told that it was normal for the skin to become a trifle reddened during the process.

When Debbie's mask was removed, not only did her face appear red, it felt decidedly irritated. Debbie remembered her mother telling her "you have to suffer for beauty," and besides, she was too embarrassed to leave. The expert put a moisturizer on Debbie's face. She said it would cool it down, and it did, and by the time Debbie left the salon, with a cosmetic makeover, she felt fine. So fine, in fact, that she listened to the salesperson recommend the following products: an anti-aging cream because "you can never start too soon"; an eye cream and a treatment product, a night cream, the moisturizer, and a toner "to close the large pores on your nose." She said she definitely needed something to close her pores.

Debbie bought two creams, an astringent, and the scrub. It cost her $134, and she left the store.

By the time she reached her office, underneath the makeover, Debbie's face was beginning to burn and her eyes were itching. She lasted until she got home that evening, and then she washed everything off. When she finished rinsing her face, she noticed small irritated patches had formed on her cheeks. They were red and dry looking. The following evening the patches were still there, and a week or so later they had company. Small whiteheads had formed on Debbie's nose and chin.

"When I looked in the mirror, I looked as though I had spots. I was a mess and didn't know what to do. I lasted that way for another day before I finally made an appointment with a dermatologist. He gave me a prescription for some pills, a lotion for the dry scaly patches, and a mild anti-acne-type medication for the whiteheads. My appointment with him cost over $100. I can't really blame the company that did the facial. I guess I should have known that I had sensitive skin and that I was prone to acne. The dermatologist said that there were several emollients and other ingredients in the anti-aging product that might spell disaster for my skin type. He felt that the reddened patches were caused by sensitivity to one of several other ingredients, possibly fragrance."

Debbie's experience is an extreme example of how a naive and badly informed consumer can be disappointed by the skin care industry.

In Debbie's case, she probably needed a more sophisticated skin care program than the one she was on. She needed a maintenance program for the oily areas on her nose and chin, and she needed a light moisturizer for the skin on her cheeks and around her eyes that was beginning to wrinkle. Because she had sensitive skin, Debbie will always have to be particularly careful about avoiding ingredients that might prove irritating.

She definitely did not *need* an expensive anti-aging cream. Her skin was too oily, and she was still too young. The products that were used on Debbie were terrific products, but they were all wrong for her skin. An older woman with drier skin could have come away from the same procedure and been absolutely thrilled with the results.

Born more than fifty years apart, my mother-in-law and Debbie are of different generations, yet they share a common desire: Each of them wants to look her best. Perhaps it is simple vanity, but it doesn't really matter; the desire to look attractive is universal, and the search for ways to increase self-beautification is as old as humanity itself. Unfortunately it has always been fraught with confusion as well as a few dangers. More than one Ancient Egyptian woman was carried off to her eternal tomb because of the mercury contained in her face powder. Today the risk of mercury poisoning, at least from cosmetic products, is relatively nonexistent. However, there are still other problems, and almost all the women I speak to are genuinely confused about what skin care means.

These are questions I've had to resolve for myself, and, appropriately, many of the women I speak to ask me what products I use and what I do to take care of my skin. My little regimen is not necessarily one that I recommend for anyone else. However, it works for me and for my skin type at this point in my life, and I think it gives a good sense of how I mix and match expensive, moderate, and inexpensive products.

My Skin Care History

As a teenager and young woman, I used next to nothing. I was fortunate as a teenager because I didn't have acne. However, I had freckles. I thought they were ugly, and they embarrassed me no end. When I was still a little girl, my father tried to make me laugh by telling me that my freckles were a result of a freak accident. He said when I was just a toddler I had been standing near a screen door, and a large paint truck went past. In this story, my nose was pressed up against the screen, and as the truck careened past, a large container of paint broke open and splashed onto the door and me.

I think I hated that explanation more than anything.

In any event, while many of my friends were smearing their faces with anti-acne preparations, I was cutting open lemons and fruitlessly, so to speak, trying to bleach my face white.

Lemons and Camay soap were all that I used on my face until I was in my twenties. Then I began using a pH-balanced soap called Lowila to wash my face and started using a moisturizer. The products I used then were Ultima's CHR Nite Cream Concentrate at night and an Elizabeth Arden moisturizer during the day. When I was in my mid-thirties, I switched to Lancôme Progrès.

Like many women, I was not too bright when it came to the sun, and in my early thirties, I spent too much time in direct sunlight. This was before sunblocks became popular, and in those years the desired look was a deep tan. So I used whatever suntan products gave me the deepest tan. Consequently, I suffered some sun damage, although it is not really visible to the naked eye.

About five years ago, a friend suggested that I try a moisturizer marketed by La Prairie, a well-known skin care company. La Prairie had a promotion soon after that, and I got a few free samples from a local department store. I found that I liked the product, and I received several compliments on the condition of my skin. Right now, this is what I use.

In the morning, I don't use soap on my face. Instead, I wash my face with a facecloth that has been rinsed in tepid water. Then I splash my face about ten or fifteen times. While it is still damp, I apply my moisturizer. Currently I am alternating between two—La Prairie Skin Conditioner, which costs almost $50 for one ounce, and Complex 15 lotion, which costs about $7 for eight ounces. By alternating the two creams, I find that I can stretch them both out for a full year.

I also use eye cream under my makeup during the day. I don't use eye cream at night because I find that it makes my eyes puffy. I use La Prairie eye cream, also about $50. Again, I use it very sparingly and replace it about once a year.

I probably should wash my face again in the middle of the day, but most of the time I don't until I remove my makeup and go to bed. At night, I do use soap. My favorite is still Lowila. It is a pH-balanced soap manufactured by Westwood Labs and it costs around $2.19 a bar. In the winter sometimes I switch to Cetaphil lotion.

Before I go to bed, I apply Capture, a skin care product manufactured by Christian Dior. It is quite expensive and costs $65 an ounce. A bottle lasts me about three months.

Approximately twice a week, I exfoliate my skin with a Buf-Puf (gentle texture). It should be used for a very short time—in my case, about thirty seconds of circular motion does it. Exfoliation gets rid of the dead skin cells and speeds up the process of cell renewal. You can buy one in a package for approximately $3.25. If you wash it out carefully, and let it dry, it should last for at least three months.

Once a week, I polish my skin with oatmeal. I keep a tin of oatmeal in the bathroom, and I pour some onto my hand, wet it, and scrub it around my face. Then I rinse carefully and apply moisturizer. I think the oatmeal gives the skin a smooth, shiny texture that I like. The oatmeal, obviously, costs pennies.

I don't get professional facials, and the mask I use most often is one I make at home and apply about once a week. I combine one egg with a tablespoon of honey and a tablespoon of cod liver oil. I smear this over my face and leave it on until it dries. Then I rinse it off with tepid water. This mask, obviously, would be too rich for someone with oily skin, and I don't recommend it for all skin types, but it works for me. When I was younger, my skin was normal to mildly oily, but right now, because my skin has matured, it has become drier. However, I still prefer moisturizers that feel lighter.

During the summer, my skin sometimes gets greasy. When that happens, I use an alcohol-free toner/astringent about two or three times a week. My department store had a special on Lancôme products recently, and I got Tonique Douceur, which was discounted to $8.79 for five ounces. I rarely use more than one bottle of toner in a year.

I usually use Vaseline Intensive Care as a body and hand lotion. I would imagine that I go through a bottle every six weeks or so. It is less expensive in larger sizes, but I get the fifteen-ounce size because I keep a container near the kitchen sink as well as one in the bathroom, and the bulkier (albeit less expensive) container takes up too much space. The price the last time I bought it was $2.79.

There are only two rules that I follow absolutely.

1. I use a moisturizer at all times, under all conditions.

2. I use a sunscreen whenever there is even a remote possibility that I will be in the sun. I choose my SPF number depending upon the circumstances. If I am going to play tennis for an hour on a court that is partially shaded, I use an 8. For a day at the beach, I choose a 15 or higher. I usually use a sunscreen made by Westwood because they have a selection I like, and I find the bottle convenient. It costs approximately $4.95 for a four-ounce bottle. Because my husband and I spend time in Florida with his mother each year, and because I spend a certain amount of time in outdoor activities, I buy about eight bottles of sunscreen yearly: three bottles with an SPF of 4 for summer activities such as walking on the street or driving; three bottles with an SPF of 8 for most activities in the sun; two bottles with an SPF of 15 for whenever I'm on a beach.

I estimate that I spend approximately $480 a year on skin care, or $40 a month. To some people this may seem excessive; to others it seems really low. What is used on my skin is based upon my needs at this time, and my pocketbook. As you can see, the products I needed and used changed as my skin changed.

Evaluating Your Skin to Create an Effective Skin Care Program

Protecting your skin is important, and here's why. Along with the physiological benefits to be gained from a good skin care program, there are innumerable ways in which well-cared-for skin can increase a woman's confidence and self-esteem. Today the average woman is going to live past seventy, so she will be staring at her reflection in the mirror for a long time. Trust me, she'll be happier if she likes what she sees.

You don't need to spend a fortune to get optimal skin care results. However, you do have to disregard hardsell techniques and decide for yourself what you want and need. These decisions should be based upon: *you* and what you want and need; and *the marketplace* and what is available.

The first and most important factor is *you.*

1. *Your* skin type. There is no way around this: Everything from how you clean your face to what you use before you go to bed should be based upon a clear understanding of what is best for your skin type.

2. *Your* age. More is known now about how skin ages; this new information should be taken into account when you make your purchasing decisions.
3. *Your* pocketbook. I understand that some women simply don't care how much they spend, but even they want products that make them look better, not worse. High ticket price doesn't guarantee anything and sometimes the best results are achieved by spending less.
4. *Your* lifestyle. Do you live in a part of the country where the air is extra dry or usually humid? Do you work in an office that is always overheated and lacks humidity? Do you spend an unusual number of hours in an airplane? Do you spend hours in the sun playing tennis? Are you an avid skier? Is it impractical for you to wash your face more than twice a day? All of these factors should be considered when making skin care purchasing decisions.

The second factor is *the marketplace.*

If you don't take the time to find out what's available, you can't possibly make well-informed choices. Too often we make decisions based solely upon what we see in the magazines. I'm not knocking the companies that advertise, but there are many others who do not spend as much on advertising whose products are just as effective, and less expensive. In some instances, you may even prefer them.

This book is designed to help the skin care consumer decide what she truly wants and needs in the way of skin care. I hope that it will help you get the most from the products available to you while avoiding some of the common pitfalls, including allergic-type reactions, cosmetic acne, and a dressing table cluttered with little-used, and very expensive, products that haven't fulfilled your expectations. I truly believe in good skin care, but I really believe that it is not necessary for the average woman to spend a fortune to get the results she wants.

Granted that the problems of the skin care consumer seem small when placed next to the national debt or the nuclear arms race. However, at seven in the morning, when you are facing your image in the bathroom mirror, you'll feel much better about yourself if you can say to yourself, "My skin looks terrific today!" And that's what this book is all about.

2

Manipulative Sales Techniques and Why They Work

A couple of years ago, *The New York Times* ran an article in its science section with the headline "Dislike of Own Body Found Common Among Women." Running in bold type under the headline was the statement, "Men Tend to See Themselves as Just About Perfect." This article summarized the findings of several studies, all of which concluded that women tend to be negatively unrealistic about the way they look. One of the researchers commented on the way in which women compare themselves, usually unfavorably, with the models and actresses whose faces they find in advertisements and in the movies. From my experience as a beauty consultant, I believe this is true.

Because I am so often exposed to the average woman's attitude about her appearance, I think about this article often. So many of the women I speak to are concerned about how they look. All over America, women—old, young, single, married, divorced—look at the faces of the models in current magazines, look at themselves in the bathroom mirror, and wonder whether they can change anything about their appearance that will make them seem more perfect. Some want to look younger and others, believe it or not, want to look older. Some want to cover spots and pimples and blemishes, others want to hide pores and wrinkles and sags.

These women, and I am one of them, are ideal targets for the cosmetics industry, an industry that, by definition, relies not only on women's insecurities, but also on their unrealistic concepts of how they should look.

I have no idea why so many women, including myself, are so often afflicted with a desire for personal perfection, and it doesn't matter whether you blame it on hormones or conditioning, or societal and sociological pressures. The fact is that much of the marketing strategy of the cosmetics industry is based on the premise that the average woman can be convinced that she needs to "do something about the way she looks."

I'm not saying that the cosmetics and skin care industry created the type of psychology that responds to skin care ads promising perfection, but they sure do everything they can to exacerbate it and capitalize on it.

From the time she is old enough to read, the budding feminine consumer is bombarded with messages telling her that beauty is a valuable commodity. When she stares at television advertisements and sees all the standardly beautiful and traditionally garbed women portraying young mothers and junior executives with Rolex watches, she can't help wondering whether she will ever be good-looking enough to make it in the cold, cruel competitive world and whether she should start thinking about "doing something" about the way she looks.

Where It Starts: Teenage Makeovers and Other Media Messages

The other day while I was visiting a friend, the phone rang, and my friend found herself involved in a long, complicated conversation with an electrician. To keep myself busy while she pleaded with him to find time to install a ceiling fixture, I started to thumb through a few teenage magazines left on the table by her thirteen-year-old daughter.

Wow! No wonder women get so confused. With a few notable exceptions, the editorial content, all directed at an adolescent female market, was supportive and constructive. Article after article advised the young readers to maintain their sense of self, to not be intimidated by their social environment, to develop a strong sense of healthy independence, etc., etc., etc.

The notable exceptions were the beauty pieces, particularly the "make-overs," some of which were on girls as young as thirteen. If I manage to repress my old-fashioned notion that a thirteen-year-old should still be thinking about doll houses, I am willing to consider the possibility that she might want to think about a look for "starting out." But why would any thirteen-year-old need a makeover? Isn't it confusing for a young girl to be told to recognize her own sense of self-worth at the same time that it is being suggested that she make herself over?

However, all of this makeover advice is not as confusing as the advertising. Here's where teenagers are told—in full-page spreads—that every-one needs to change her hair color (even temporarily) every now and then, that a certain foundation makeup is more like "perfecting your skin than making it up," or that "if you've always felt you had puny lashes . . ." you should try Lash Out Extending Mascara.

To me the average young reader is going to get three messages loud and clear from these ads—all of which, by the way, feature absolutely gorgeous models. The first: Beauty is very, very important. The second: The young reader will probably need to change something about herself if she wants to secure a place in the glamorous adult world. If she believed all the advertisements, she might think that she needs to change her hair color, to perfect her skin, and to extend her eyelashes. She might also need to style her hair, color her eyelids, blush her cheeks, clear her face with a product other than soap and water, and just generally shape up. The third: She needs help doing all of this, and this help is going to come from all the products featured on those slick glossy pages.

As women, all of us have received these messages from early adolescence. We are not perfect, and we should change our eyes, change our hair, change our mouth, change our complexion . . . in short, change our faces.

This message is a highly charged one. It preys on a woman's insecurity, and whenever a woman feels less than perfect, which for many of us is more often than we like to admit, it makes us susceptible to the underlying promises in the cosmetics advertisements, the promises that tell us that greater desirability and physical beauty are possible with the right cosmetic products. These are the "buy" messages that are supposed to make us want to rush out and try every product now on the market.

Unfortunately, when we respond to the "buy" messages in skin care advertisements, we forget about shopping in a way that makes sense, and we are vulnerable to impractical, expensive, and silly purchases that don't satisfy our needs.

Responding to the "buy" message in skin care promotions is an easy thing to do, and a mood that I think most women identify with. We walk into a department store cosmetics department, stop at a counter, and suddenly we are walking out of the store clutching a shopping bag containing a few outrageously expensive skin care items. When we look at them and see what we spent, we tend to try to rationalize our purchases. Typically a woman will tell herself that she was "doing something good for herself," and that she deserves the best skin care products.

Don't misunderstand. I don't for a moment question any woman's right to treat herself to excellent skin care. What I question is whether or not these purchases reflect either good judgment, or whether the typical skin consumer is getting the products she should have for her skin. All too often what happens is that a woman becomes discouraged and disappointed by what she buys and gives up. When a product doesn't deliver, there is a tendency to hesitate before trying anything else. The average woman who spent a hundred dollars or more for a couple of one-ounce containers that don't work the way she hoped has a tendency to resist spending more money and resists trying anything else—until the next time she is in a cosmetics department and that old urge for change hits.

There is another problem here, and I think we have to admit it if we are going to stop being manipulated by skin care advertisements. As women, most of us want to be beautiful. As intelligent, sensitive adults who honestly believe that "beauty is only skin deep," many of us are embarrassed by self-vanity. This conflict makes us confused, and emotional, and we never develop a sensible, practical way of dealing with skin care purchases. We don't develop sensible skin care budgets, we don't analyze our needs, and we don't comparison shop. Instead, we often rely upon whim and impulse, allowing our emotions to turn us into impractical and ill-informed consumers. There is a right way and a wrong way to make skin care purchases. Treating buying as though it is an emotional decision is always the wrong way.

When Skin Care Products Become an Emotional Decision—A History

Janet is forty-seven years old. She has a graduate degree in English and a successful public relations business. She is divorced and she has successfully raised a son to responsible adulthood. Yet she is insecure about shopping for cosmetics and skin care products. She has always been a skin care consumer, and she has always made impulse purchases. The emotional appeal of a product is what comes first.

The fact is, I'm torn. If I spend a lot of money, I feel as though I am being "taken"—as if I'm a fool for believing all the stuff in the ads and department stores. If I don't spend enough money, then I think that I'm not doing everything I can for my appearance.

I have a long history of buying the wrong lipstick and eyeshadows (this is interesting because I have never worn eyeshadow—I just buy it thinking some day I will), but where I really waste money is with face cream. I love face cream. I have always loved face cream. But I've always felt that I'm doing the wrong thing, and I'm really not sure what to do. Recently I was in a department store, and the cosmetics salesperson told me I should do something about my pores. Well, I don't know what to do about my pores. I feel the same way now that I did when I was fourteen years old.

Then (which was back in the 1950s), every Saturday afternoon, I would wash my hair and set it in bobby pins. While I was waiting for it to dry, I would give myself a facial. I had read about facials in one of my mother's magazines and immediately decided that they were imperative to my social success.

In any event, often my best friend would come over and we had a little routine worked out. We would smear Pond's dry skin cream on our faces. Then we would wipe it off with tissues and lay back, our faces covered with cucumber slices. My friend had read somewhere that cucumber was "the best."

Finally we would finish up with *the mask*. I don't remember the name of the product, but it had been advertised in a magazine, and my friend and I chipped in to buy it at the department store in the nearest big city. To this day I remember how ravishing the advertising copy on the label implied, if not actually promised, that you would look if you used the mask. I think I related it somehow to stories about movie stars and the masks then used. In any event, we would smear on the mask, wait for it to dry, and take it off. I still remember my anticipation at taking the mask off. Every time. The same thrill. I'm not sure what I expected, but certainly something wonderful. I would look in the mirror and stare and try to see what had happened. To me, nothing had happened. It was the same old face. Instead of questioning the product, of course I questioned my perception. I decided the results were so subtle that they were not immediately discernable to someone who was accustomed to looking at her own face and that I looked at my face in the mirror so often that I just couldn't see what had happened. But when I looked at my friend, nothing changed on her face either. Nonetheless we continued this routine until the contents of the mask jar were dry and crumbled on the bottom.

Now that I'm an adult, I'm really no wiser. I still look at the advertisements and feel impelled to run out and buy. I still rush home and throw the latest glop on my face. I still expect a miracle. I still look in the mirror, and I still don't see a difference. The only thing that's changed is the price tag. Now, the cosmetics that appeal to me are outrageously expensive. Recently I wandered into a department store and wandered out less than thirty minutes later and more than $130 poorer. I have no idea why I always do this.

I think I have a fairly good idea why Janet so often ends up with the wrong products. Janet, who always wants to look her best, is very aware of her appearance. Rightly or wrongly, she has been conditioned to make a connection between the way she looks and the way her skin looks. But Janet doesn't know how to manage her skin or what products and skin care regimen will work for her, and she doesn't know how to find out except through trial and error. She is, consequently, very responsive and vulnerable to the hardsell "buy" messages that are part and parcel of skin care promotions.

The Hard Sell—What Skin Care Consumers Are Up Against

Advertisers use language to manipulate consumers. They know we are all somewhat infatuated with ourselves, and they take advantage of this self-interest. Nowhere is this more obvious than when they advertise.

One of the primary reasons why cosmetics companies are so aggressive in trying to get you, the consumer, to try their product is that a great deal of the research done in recent years shows that the cosmetics and skin care consumer is brand-loyal.

I have seen this personally many times. A woman may start out using only one product from a particular skin care line, but if she is satisfied with it, when she goes to replace it she will purchase a couple of other products from the line, and so it goes. Eventually, the consumer may end up using the entire line. And anyone who finds herself so devoted to a product line that she is buying soap, cleansing creams, scrubs, astringents, masks, eye creams, neck creams, moisturizers, body lotions, hand lotions, anti-aging substances, etc., may be spending much more than is necessary.

As any woman who has flipped the pages of a magazine knows, cosmetics companies spend lots and lots of money on advertising, and skin care products get a lion's share of the advertising dollar. There is a reason why manufacturers do so much magazine advertising. In 1984, *Savvy* did a study of cosmetics use, and when the respondents were asked where they found out about new products, fragrances, or colors, 69.5 percent replied "magazines" and 53.8 percent replied "advertising." Skin care manufacturers know that advertising is what sells their products, and they spend their money accordingly.

In the late 1980s, for example, annual advertising expenditure for skin care products was well over $122,000,000. About $50,000,000 of that money was spent on magazine advertising; another $68,000,000 (give or take a mil) was spent on television ads; and the rest went for newspaper supplements and radio.

The big spender was Procter & Gamble, which dished out over $19,000,000 to advertise Oil of Olay. Other heavy advertisers included Lancôme ($8,000,000), Pond's ($6,000,000), Estée Lauder ($2,788,100 for Night Repair), and Clinique ($1,133,900 for facial lotion and soap).

This $122,000,000 skin care figure does not include the $84,000,000 spent on medicated skin products such as Clearasil, Chap Stick, Noxzema Medicated Skin Cream, and sunscreen products. Noxell was the big spender here—$8,000,000+ on Noxzema Medicated Skin Cream alone.

How does advertising for skin care products compare with spending on other types of cosmetics?

Take a look at one year's worth of estimated advertising dollars for:

Facial makeup	$53,000,000+
Fragrances	$115,000,000+
Lip and eye products	$68,000,000+
Manicure products	$94,000,000+
Medicated skin products	$84,000,000+
Men's products	$82,000,000+
Shampoos and rinses	$155,000,000+
Skin care products	$122,000,000+

If you count the number of advertising pages in most women's magazines, you will see what these figures mean. Every few pages, there is a shampoo ad, but running a close second is the number of pages devoted to skin care products. Can you guess which magazines have the greatest share of the skin care advertising dollar? *Vogue,*

Glamour, Cosmopolitan, Harper's Bazaar, and *Good Housekeeping* are some of the most popular.

The ads you read are somewhat determined by the magazines you buy, and the magazines, in turn, are clearly directed toward specific readership groups. While adolescent women read *Seventeen* and other youth-oriented periodicals, more mature readers might prefer *Harper's Bazaar.* Young single women read *Cosmopolitan, Mademoiselle,* and *Glamour.* Married women tend to read *Redbook, Good Housekeeping,* and *Ladies' Home Journal.* And so it goes.

Advertisers are interested in what you read. Studies of income levels, education levels, age levels, etc., are available for most of the women-oriented magazines. These studies are used by advertisers, including skin care manufacturers, when they decide where and how to pitch their products.

When a young woman picks up *Seventeen,* she sees ads by companies such as Noxzema and Clearasil directed at adolescent skin problems, and when a more mature woman picks up *Harper's Bazaar,* she is more likely to see ads for Night Repair and Oil of Olay.

But the underlying message to the reader, no matter what her age, is always the same, "You need this product to help make you perfect."

Pimples and Wrinkles: The Two Major Skin "Imperfections"

When the average woman worries about "perfection" she is usually considering more than just physical beauty. She is worrying about being a perfect friend, a perfect lover, a perfect wife, a perfect mother, a perfect daughter, a perfect 10. She also worries about being perfect in her profession, perfect in the kitchen, perfect in bed. When we read magazines and newspapers we see that even celebrities and other women who seemed overwhelmingly beautiful to start out with are having face lifts, chin lifts, and tummy tucks.

In our personal and emotional lives, it is often difficult to define perfect. With our skin, it's not so complicated, and perhaps this is part of the appeal of skin care products. Perfect skin means no pimples and no wrinkles. Which one you worry about usually depends upon your age.

The Pimple Pitch

Whether you call them comedones, blackheads, whiteheads, milia, or pimples, they spell out blemish, for all the world to see. And teenage girls (and boys) worry about them, along with everything else they worry about. However, there is a difference in what happens when boys worry and when girls worry. Teenage boys actually have as many cases of acne as teenage girls and go to as many dermatologists, but they are not as likely as young women to get hooked on the skin care game, and few major marketing efforts are aimed at their skin care worries. Just about every time a young woman picks up a magazine, in an amazing number of articles and advertisements she will be reminded of her blemishes and told about all the various products she can buy to help get rid of pimples, prevent pimples, etc.

Many young women also get the impression that pimples are associated with dirty skin, and, since so many cleansing products are available for teenage skin, they sometimes come away with the impression that they can "scrub" the pimples away.

It is estimated that close to 80 percent of American teenagers have some form of acne at one time or another. Keeping that statistic in mind, it is easy to see why the young female skin care consumer is a prime candidate for any and all cleansing products.

The Zits Nightmare—Buying into "Pimples"

When I met Greta a few years ago, she was a very pretty woman with amazingly dry skin. She was in her mid-forties and had the driest skin I had ever seen—and the cleanest. When I suggested that she needed to replace moisture, she told me that her skin was too oily. She said that her whole family suffered from oily skin and that she didn't want to run the risk of pimples. While I tried to convince her to buy a humidifier and start using moisturizer, I also asked her how her attitude toward her skin had evolved. Here's what she told me:

> When I was a teenager, I was obsessed with not getting what my mother referred to as a zit. My older sister always got pimples, and it seemed to me as if every surface in our house had a little tube of some ointment or another and a mirror. Carol also had zit stories, like: "Let me tell you about the time I got the zit on the end of my nose the day

before I had to sing the solo in choir, and when I got up, I knew all
everybody could think about was the zit on my nose."

Small wonder that I, too, spent an inordinate amount of time
thinking about pimples. I picked at my skin and examined it every
chance I got. Every time I had a major event I worried every time that
I would wake up in the morning and discover zits. Ycch.

The day before the big football game, I worried; the week before the
senior prom, I worried; the month before my wedding, I worried.

To this day I still have nightmares in which I look in a mirror and
discover a little sea of pimples on my forehead.

Greta, who washed her face at least three times a day with oatmeal soap
and a rough washcloth and used a clay mask three times a week and an
alcohol toner, is a good example of a woman who has purposely dried out
her skin in order to avoid greasy "stuff."

But there is another end of this spectrum.

Wrinkle Fever

Margo is an amazingly beautiful forty-five-year-old woman. Tall, slender,
elegant, and lovely, she has naturally silver blonde hair, perfect teeth,
perfect features, and a lilting British accent. When she was still in her
twenties, she vowed that as she got older, she would do whatever she
could to prevent wrinkles and maintain her beauty. Many of the women
I spoke to who were compulsive skin care consumers started out with a
fear of pimples. Margo is no exception.

As a teenager, I worried about pimples. I thought I had acne. In
reality I had two large pimples that would recur once a month; they
seemed to be connected to my menstrual cycle. But I started thinking
about ways to get rid of them and ways to cover them.

At first I bought very little. My family didn't have much money so I
would improvise. I followed instructions in magazines and made
egg-white masks, and I used witch hazel as a toner to dry out my skin.

Then when my skin started to get too dry, I started using egg yolks
and fresh milk and dairy cream to wash my face. This was still before
I was old enough to work and earn money for skin care products.

As soon as I was working on my own, I started spending money on
cosmetics and skin care products. I would walk into department store
cosmetics departments and immediately get intimidated.

The salespeople would indicate they thought I could be prettier if I
did the right thing for my skin. I interpreted this to mean that there

was something wrong with me, and, more often than not, I would buy what they recommended.

Also, and I'm ashamed to admit this, but it's true—I thought I wanted a career and wouldn't have time to think about marriage until my late twenties. I worried that if I waited that long I wouldn't be able to compete in the crazy dating market unless I looked younger than my age. So I started thinking about wrinkles in my early twenties, and I've been thinking about them ever since.

At one time or another, I think I have used every product line made. I used Lancôme exclusively for a while; then I used Elizabeth Arden because I would go there for facials. Then I've used La Prairie, Orlane, CHR, Glycel, Estée Lauder, Clinique. You name it, I've tried it.

At first I was a pushover because I was insecure; now, I'm a pushover because I look in the mirror and remember what I used to see, and I try to recapture it. So I'll buy anything . . . within reason. I have often bought a whole line of products and let them get rancid because I didn't like them, or they made me break out. Don't forget, I still have mildly oily skin, and some of this stuff is very rich. I know this, and yet I buy it and then I'm furious at myself.

I also get facials at private salons, and, here, I have learned. I'm very careful to start out by saying clearly that I just want a facial and I don't want any products. Because I don't want the person giving facials to feel that I have taken too much time without buying anything, I tend to overtip and give generous Christmas gifts.

The facials often make my skin terrific, and give me a little touch of the past, a glimpse of a look that I remember having.

I'm the first to admit that I'm buying hope. Does anything really work? I have to say yes. A lot of things make my skin look better. And, then, a lot of things just make me break out.

I like to feel that I'm doing everything I can to keep my looks, so I don't resent spending money on all of these products. What I resent is my own stupidity in not being able to say no and that I'm so easily manipulated and let it work on my mind.

Margo has always been so beautiful that I couldn't imagine how she could feel intimidated at the beauty counter. In every other area of her life, Margo is a remarkably cost-conscious and amazingly practical woman, but because she is totally unrealistic about the way she looks she is a completely impractical beauty consumer.

Being a Practical Skin Care Consumer

I love skin care products, but I hate the sales pitch, the confusing advertising, and the high prices. If a woman wants to look her best, there is no substitute for beautiful skin, but before she can evaluate what products, if any, are going to help her achieve that goal, she has to know what's sold, and how it's sold.

3

How Skin Care Products Are Sold

In Department Stores

The hardsell "buy" messages are heard loudest in the large department store cosmetics department; here's where the pressure is really on. A cosmetics department can be very important to a department store because the larger companies tend to spend money on advertisements and promotion. These, in turn, help entice consumers into the store. When a consumer who is responding to such a sales promotion visits the cosmetics counter, there is a very good possibility that she will linger and go to other departments, hence increasing sales throughout the store.

The New York Bloomingdale's cosmetics department probably provides the best example of a somewhat overwhelming skin care sales pitch.

Bloomies, N.Y.—You Are There!

Brilliantly lit, extravagantly fitted out, and awesomely glamorous, Bloomingdale's cosmetics department is an example of the skin care industry at its exciting best and high-pressured worst.

Take a walk with me through the department: Come in the Lexington Avenue entrance, walk through costume jewelry, past hats, up the stairs, and you are in the cosmetics department. Before you arrive, you smell it. Beautiful young men and women stand at the top of the stairs waiting to offer passersby a perfume hit. Today the fragrance of choice appears to be Elizabeth Taylor's Passion, and one of the elegantly dressed men is walking from side to side across the top two stairs, spraying whenever he finds a willing wrist. There seems to be no way to avoid either him or the perfume's ubiquitous mist.

At the top of the stairs, I pause for a second to get my bearings.

"Would you like a free makeover today?" asks a woman wearing a lab coat. I see she is working at a Chanel counter. Behind her is the space that Adrien Arpel has carved out—there a woman seated on a stool is having her face worked on by another lab-coated woman; it seems they are also offering free makeovers. I say no to the Chanel representative and walk a few feet down the aisle. I stop again, just to figure out where I am, and a Lancôme rep is with me. They, too, are offering makeovers.

I continue on, shaking my head no. At the next counter, I glance at a piece of promotional literature for a relatively new company, Intelligent Skincare. By the time I pick up the brochure the salesperson is there. . . . "No thanks," I say. "Just browsing."

Half a second later, I'm at the Prescriptives Counter, where there is a large promotional piece with the heading NEWS TEAM PRESCRIPTIVES BULLETIN. Prescriptives is an Estée Lauder product, but the Prescriptives line has its own counter. As a matter of fact, if you were to measure power by the space allotted to each company, Estée Lauder would definitely be the queen at Bloomingdale's. When it comes to territory, the company has a distinct edge. It seems as though everywhere you look there is a Lauder representative.

If a company has more space, it usually means that it is the store's top seller. In a few stores, the cosmetics company actually buys space, but in most of them their financial contribution is best seen in their advertising and promotion budgets. The cosmetics company may, for example, guarantee a certain amount of advertising or promotion dollar in return for the larger space. Remember, successful products mean that there will be more customers in the store.

When I stop to read the Prescriptives Line Away promotional material, the saleswoman approaches me.

"Do you know about the free radical theory?" she asks. I am about to reply, but she continues on, "Well, free radicals are formed from UV rays. . . ."

Because I know I am not going to buy anything, I feel too guilty to allow her to continue, and I quickly move on. As I walk, I can't help but be amused at the way in which the free radical theory of aging has been taken on by the cosmetics industry. That's when I took a good look at Bloomingdale's cosmetics department in its entirety. It had changed, and I hadn't even noticed. Nearly everywhere I looked, I saw a cosmetics company employee wearing a white lab coat; there was a definite emphasis on science.

La Prairie, for example, had a small room, fitted out almost like a small clinic. Clinique, which had a great deal of open space with an inviting-looking white table, even had a sign that said "Clinique Lab Room." And, of course, there was the "Clinique Computer," which added to the scientific flavor.

Most of the salespeople were young women, but there were more men than I remembered, including several mature-looking men. At the Biotherm counter, it looked as though there were more lab-coated men than women. I whizzed past Clarins, Germaine Monteil, Madeleine Mono, Orlane, and Revlon, but I stopped at the Frances Denney counter to pick up some literature. Big mistake! The representative was with me before I could even reach for the promotional material.

Some of the companies that sell at Bloomingdale's have more than one space. Christian Dior, for example, had a counter in the middle of the floor as well as another separate space along the rim of the department. Here, there were at least six lab-coated men and women working, and the three men looked more mature than is customary, and slightly professorial. There were two main attractions at the Dior space: the makeover computer, which gives color printouts with suggested makeup, and Capture, the skin care product that features liposomes. The Dior representatives were stopping anyone who hesitated and telling her about Capture and the computer makeover. They were also offering a trial size of the product with every Capture purchase, saying that the purchase could be returned if the customer wasn't satisfied with the results from the sample size.

Shiseido had several women working at their counter, selling as well as directing potential customers to another floor where the Shiseido computer was set up for a special promotion.

And, as I said, every time I hesitated, a salesperson was there. "Can I show you?" "Can I tell you?" "Can I help you?" Estée Lauder had a promotion—purchase $15 worth of products and you get a free gift. Since Lauder has so much space in Bloomingdale's, it was difficult to pass through the center aisle without running into a representative displaying the gift, a travel kit with sample products. Elizabeth Arden also had a promotion. Their gift: sample products with a $12.95 purchase.

The total time I spent in the Bloomingdale's cosmetics department was under seven minutes. In that time, I was approached by eighteen salespeople. I truly wanted to spend more time, ask more questions, and just generally browse, but it was all too overwhelming.

The Cosmetics Salesperson as True Believer

When you walk through a cosmetics department, take a look around. The floor is filled with people who are getting a commission on what you buy. Let me warn you, if something catches your eye, and you stop even for the briefest moment, you will be approached by a salesperson who is often an employee of the skin care manufacturer, not of the department store, and is usually trained by the cosmetics manufacturer, not the store. Because they are monetarily rewarded on sales, they are anxious to sell the most expensive products, in the largest quantities.

The cosmetics employees behind the counters, and wandering the floor, know their business; they are there to sell. You, in turn, are supposed to be there to buy. Try to browse, or comparison shop, and you feel like a penny-pinching interloper and a misdirected misfit. The atmosphere in the department, combined with the attitude of the cosmetics salesperson, makes most women feel as though they are either buyers and, hence, belongers or failed freshman sorority rejects.

The cosmetics salesperson is perhaps the most powerful department store selling tool. When I first began buying cosmetics, it seemed to me that the typical salesperson was an intimidating middle-aged woman who wore a lot of makeup and had an infuriatingly condescending manner. Now it seems as though the typical salesperson is a young woman with wholesome good looks and a light touch with the makeup brush. Also, there are now more men selling cosmetic products, particularly skin care.

But male, female, young, middle-aged, or mature, the cosmetics salesperson is, first and foremost, probably going to be a true believer.

I've talked to a lot of skin care employees, and it continues to astound me how totally most of them believe in the product they are selling, whichever product it is. The Shiseido salesperson thinks Shiseido is best, the Clinique salesperson thinks Clinique is the best, the Lancôme salesperson thinks Lancôme is the best, etc. Perhaps this cheerleader-like enthusiasm is the most important requirement for getting these jobs, but what really matters is the way in which this enthusiasm is conveyed to you, the consumer.

I know that when I sold cosmetics, I also believed in the product. When I ceased to believe, I was no longer effective and couldn't bring myself to push the line. This commitment to a product line is a large part of what makes the cosmetics representative such an irresistible salesperson, but the important thing for the consumer to remember is not to be overwhelmed by the salesperson's disciple-like devotion to the product. No matter how perfect the complexion or how dedicated the sales pitch, the cosmetics company salesperson is not your own personal skin care guru.

Incidentally, the skin care salesperson is usually trained by the company in both selling and understanding the company's products. This training—typically a seminar of one to three days—includes a lesson in how to diagnose skin type as well as in which of *their* products to recommend for different skins. When new products are introduced, the employees are often called back for additional training. Employees who work the computers or skin analyzers receive further training. Although the employee is given basic information about the skin, the emphasis is very much on product recommendations and sales.

Some Favorite Department Store Sales Techniques

Clinics, Labs, and Other Semiscientific Sales Techniques Probably the newest sales approach is centered on the skin care industry's desire to appear "scientific." When they first started to use phrases such as "treatment cosmetics," manufacturers discovered that women respond to the scientific approach.

In 1987 the FDA started to crack down on exaggerated skin care claims of a scientific nature. Some manufacturers have responded to this, and other stimuli, by moving the "science" out of the ads and into the department stores, where visual effects can almost create the illusion that you are walking into a laboratory as opposed to walking up to a cosmetics counter. Accentuating this semiscience atmosphere are words and phrases such as "clinic," "miniclinic," "latest technology," "skin analysis," "computerized results," "image analysis," "digitalized analysis," "micro," "lipids," "noncomedegenic," etc.

It is all designed to make you feel as though modern science and technology have worked miracles in the anti-aging department and that if you are not trying the latest product, you are going to be the only woman left in America with a lined face. These are very powerful sales techniques that work on a subliminal as well as conscious level, and the consumer should not be hoodwinked into thinking that the sales representative, who, remember, has received only minimal training in the science of skin care, is the purveyor of scientific gospel. In other words, watch out!

Low-Cost Facials with Free Gift Several companies pursue this method of getting new business. Here's how it's done: The skin care company places an ad in the local newspaper telling the consumer that low-cost facials will be available at the company's cosmetics counter. The ad gives the days and hours when this service will be given, lists a price—usually under $25—and asks the consumer either to call for an appointment or to stop by at the cosmetics counter at an appropriate time. More often than not, the ad promises a small gift such as a makeup tote as well as several small samples of the company's skin care products.

My friend Julie recently had a facial at the Adrien Arpel counter at Saks in New York. Here's her experience:

A friend saw the ad and made an appointment for both of us. When we arrived, three women were having their faces worked on. The women who were giving the facials were all young and had beautiful skin. The one who did my face said that she had worked for several other companies but had recently come to Arpel and liked their products. When I was there, the women receiving facials were all over forty and didn't seem to be particularly experienced cosmetics or skin care buyers.

The young woman who worked on my face was very deft, although I must admit that the machine used in the cleansing process irritated my skin. When I told her that, she stopped immediately. No one asked me my skin type or made any attempt to find it out. I was told that my skin lacked moisture and it was suggested that I might want to try several of the company's products for dry skin. She also put cream on my hands and put them in gloves while she worked. That was nice.

Even though there was very little pressure applied, I still felt foolish about walking away with the gift, a nice little cosmetics bag with several free samples without buying more products. I bought the little vials with collagen and I got a moisturizer and some eye cream. All in all, including the cost of the facial, I spent close to $150. I liked the collagen product, but the moisturizer I chose was much too light for my skin, which is dry. I gave it to my daughter, however, and she absolutely loves it. Says it is perfect for her. I loved the Honey and

Almond Scrub, but so did my husband. I let him try it, and that was
the end of that.

I was glad I had the experience, but I don't think I would do it
again. I always walk away from this sort of thing more insecure than
when I started, and I always spend more money than I want to. It's
true that my skin felt very smooth, but it didn't look any different.
However, it was smooth enough for my husband to comment on.

The product that I would go back for: the Honey and Almond
Scrub. I liked the way it made my skin feel, and I intend to buy some
more the next time I'm in a department store.

Computer Skin Analysis Doesn't that sound like fun! Computers are
the latest rage in skin analysis. Theoretically, they can analyze the texture
and condition of your skin. How much it costs depends upon how much
you buy. These computers are usually found in large department stores
in connection with a specific promotion. Traveling along with the computer are the company's experts, salespeople, and consultants trained to
use the technology and analyze the results. The customer often receives
some form of printout suggesting products from the company's skin care
line. There is sometimes a charge for the skin analysis, but it can be
applied against purchases.

Although I'm told that several companies, including Elizabeth Arden,
have skin care computers, the only one that I see regularly is the Shiseido
computer. Some of the larger department stores have a permanent instal-
lation, and the smaller ones are visited by the computer and the operators.

Shiseido uses a process they call the Replica™ Skin Diagnosis System.
Nancy, a thirty-one-year-old attorney, had this done recently in a large
department store:

> I didn't have an appointment; I was just meandering through the
> skin care department. Near the Shiseido counter, I saw a large sign
> with computer-type blowups of skin sections. Two women, both of
> whom were in their mid-twenties and beautifully made up, were
> standing near the sign and one of them approached me and asked if I
> would like to have my skin analyzed. I asked how much it cost and
> was told it was free, so I figured why not?
>
> Anyway, another very good-looking woman, in her early twenties,
> sat me down on a stool and cleaned off a section of skin on my cheek.
> She then prepared this reddish paste about the size of a fifty-cent piece;
> she said it was a nontoxic dental paste, and she put it on my left cheek
> and left it there for about two minutes.

While waiting for it to dry, she showed me photographs of computer analyses of several different types of skin. One was oily, one was dry, one was normal, one had large pores, etc. The woman said that lines show dehydration. Ideally, she said, the skin should look plumped out and that the plump areas are triangles. She said that dark holes are pores and that dry skin looks flat.

Then she peeled off the dried paste and stuck it under what looked like a microscope, and I saw the results on the computer terminal. I tried to compare my skin with the photographs I had seen earlier, but, to be perfectly frank, I couldn't tell the difference.

The woman working with me said I had large pores and oily skin. I was surprised because I always thought it was dry. However, we agreed that I might have overmoisturized, whatever that means. In any event, I agreed that my pores might be too large, and we agreed upon a skin care plan using Shiseido products. I spent a fortune.

I bought something called Cleansing Foam for $17. I bought a brush to use with it, but I don't remember what that cost. I also bought a mask for $22.50. Plus I bought some eyecream, which I really think I needed, so I'm happy about that. I'm not so happy about the price—it was $35. I also bought the skin care B–24 Day/Night for $60, but by that time who was counting?

I don't know why I bought so much. I guess I got worried about my pores and I got to feeling insecure. I looked so frumpy next to these women. On the one hand, I felt sorry for them because they had to stand around in a department store mushing cream on people's faces, but on the other hand, I felt they knew something I didn't know. They knew how to look beautiful, and I felt like a washout in that department. My reactions were really odd.

I think they were supposed to give me a little pamphlet with my skin analysis and skin care program written out, but they didn't. They did tell me that I could come back a month after trying the cleansing program and check my skin out again. I suppose I should have, but, to be perfectly frank, I was afraid I'd spend another hundred dollars. Also, to be honest, they made me feel as if my skin was so bad that it was useless for me to try anything, because my attempts were doomed to failure.

The only product I've used faithfully is the eye cream, so I can't tell whether or not any of it does anything. I never even unpacked the brush.

I think the skin analysis is a good idea, but I got the feeling that I still wasn't doing the right thing.

Nancy is right, the skin analysis is a good idea, but how successful it is, is entirely dependent upon how expert your "expert" is at evaluating the analysis. There is no way of knowing whether you are getting an accurate analysis or just an enthusiastic try.

Free Sample Product I must admit this is one of my favorite skin care "buy messages," a low-key "Here, try the product."

If a woman loves the product, she'll come back. If it's an old ho hum . . . well, that's that.

A friend of mine was recently in a department store, and she walked past the Christian Dior counter.

> I stopped for a moment at the counter, and a woman rushed up to ask me if she could help me. I was just sort of staring at all the products and I immediately said no, that I was just looking. I expected her to become annoyed and make me feel terrible about not buying. Instead, she pulled out a little sample of Capture, wrote her name on the side of the package, and said, "Try it. . . . You'll be back."
>
> "Is it wonderful?" I asked her.
>
> She pointed to her skin and said, "It has made my skin look years younger."
>
> She was obviously an older woman, but she did have beautiful skin. I took her words with a grain of salt, went home, put the sample on a shelf, and forgot about it for a few weeks until one night I ran out of my regular night cream and decided to try Capture. I tried it for the next few nights, and perhaps I'm imagining it, but my skin looks much better to me. In any event, I ran back and bought the product. I love it!

Purchase with Purchase and Gift with Purchase Two other tried-and-true promotional methods of luring new customers into the department store cosmetics department are free Gift with Purchase and Purchase with Purchase, otherwise known as GWP and PWP.

Estée Lauder probably started the whole PWP/GWP promotions. In the 1960s, when Lauder was a young company, they wanted to entice new customers, but they had a small advertising budget. This system worked, and other companies started to use the free gift with purchase technique of encouraging sales. If you buy more than $25 worth of products, for example, you will get a gift. Some of these gifts are quite nice and attractively packaged. However, they are often products you may not necessarily want to use, or the sample size, particularly if it is a body or hand lotion, is so small that it's next to useless.

Sometimes you may see these special promotions advertised; other times you become aware of them when you walk through the cosmetics department. If you stop for a moment at the counter, you will hear the salesperson's voice saying, "We have a special promotion today. . . ."

However, you may hear that voice less often. Some companies have found the gimmick expensive and are gradually tapering off. The GWP and PWP detractors say that as the gimmick has multiplied, consumers have come to take it for granted, and it has lost its effectiveness.

For most companies Gift With Purchase is preferred over Purchase with Purchase. The reason: unsold PWPs were often returned to the manufacturer, leaving the company with obsolete merchandise and lower sales than had been anticipated.

Outside the Department Store

Drug and Chain Stores

Buying in drug and chain stores is certainly favored by many women, particularly those shopping for less expensive brand name products. Here's where women go to replace their moderately priced skin care staples. In my experience, in this low-pressure, safe environment, women respond best to the brands that they have used before.

Edie, a forty-three-year-old lawyer, the mother of two teenaged daughters, is someone who regularly shops at drug/chain stores.

> There is a large Duane Reade near me, and approximately once a month or so I drop in on my way home from work and stock up. . . . I get Vaseline Intensive Care, which we all use as a hand lotion; I also buy Noxzema for one daughter who loves it and Bonne Bell Ten-O-Six lotion for the other. In the summer I get enough sunscreen for the whole family. Other products I buy here include witch hazel, my husband's shaving cream, shampoo, etc. We tend to buy the larger sizes to save money.

The woman who shops in discount drugstores rarely thinks she is spending more than she should or that she is buying products she doesn't need or want. There is a certain amount of impulse buying in response to merchandising stimuli, but the typical consumer I spoke to indicated that impulse buying was mostly confined to color cosmetics such as lipsticks or nail polish; she doesn't feel she is making extravagant or wasteful skin care purchases because most of the time she is replacing tried and true skin care products.

Although several of the products sold in these outlets, including Oil of Olay, Nivea, Noxzema, and Vaseline, are frequent advertisers, within the drug discount department there is usually no pressure whatsoever to buy, and the consumer is happily left to her own devices to wander around, picking up the products she wants. As a matter of fact, a survey done a few years back indicated that only 12 percent of drugstore shoppers reported that the cosmetics sales clerk actually helped them make a purchase.

Supermarkets

Supermarkets across the country carry a supply of skin care products such as Eucerin, Nivea, Vaseline Intensive Care, and Jergens, as well as some sunscreens. Although many of the women I spoke to said that they made some purchases at their local supermarket, most said they found it frustrating because of the limited selection. I have found that only the largest stores carry a dependable stock.

Cosmetics Boutiques

Cosmetics boutiques are found throughout the country. In the suburbs they are often located in shopping malls. In big cities, one finds them on the little streets in neighborhoods that specialize in small, personalized stores. Most often the cosmetics boutiques carry only one line of skin care products and other cosmetics. Sometimes it is a private label that is sold locally.

I am an enthusiastic advocate of some of the private-label products that I've used. Often they are not only good products, but also relatively inexpensive. However, shopping in the private-label boutiques can be an expensive experience if you buy too much. The environment often feels low-key and comfortable. You may be the only person in the shop and getting a lot of attention. This is nice, but it can lead to feelings of guilt about the attention and can cause you to make a substantial purchase. Private-label cosmetics sometimes also have a small section in larger outlets, such as drugstores.

A word of warning: The products are sometimes so reasonably priced you may be tempted to buy more than you really need.

If you want to find a private-label company, take a look in the yellow pages under Cosmetics. The private-label cosmetics will usually be the ones with the names you don't recognize. You can check them out first on the phone by asking what line of cosmetics the store carries and verifying that it is a private-label boutique.

One of the oldest established private labels is Kiehl's, which was first established as a pharmacy in 1851. Kiehl's prides itself on never advertising, relying instead on word of mouth. They have outlets throughout the United States. To find out about their product line and/or order, phone (212) 677-3171 or fax (212) 674-3544.

Another type of cosmetics boutique is one that carries a nationally franchised cosmetics label. Perhaps the best example of this is Merle Norman, which has over 2,300 outlets across the country. Merle Norman sells both cosmetic and skin care products. Whether the experience is low-key or high pressure usually depends upon the personality of the owner or beauty advisor working in the individual store. Merle Norman is a moderately priced cosmetic. Probably the most expensive product is their anti-aging cream, Luxiva Energizing Concentrate. It is $35 for one ounce. If you want to find a Merle Norman outlet, try your local phone book, or get their 800 number.

Facial Salons

I must admit that I've never had a facial, because I'm squeamish about having somebody "pick" at my face. However, I have friends who swear by facials. Pat, a thirty-nine-year-old actress, recently had one that pleased her a lot. If you've ever wondered what happens at one of these high-priced beauty establishments, here's her experience:

> All facials start pretty much the way this one did: The operator showed me into a small room, where I was instructed to lie down on a recliner and I was encouraged to remove my blouse and skirt so I would feel comfortable. She covered me with a sheet and, using a band, pulled the hair off my face.
>
> First my operator, whose name was Theresa, covered my face with a cleansing cream, which she wiped off with cotton. Then she used a lotion on my face, and again wiped it off.
>
> When she was finished with this, she used a large magnifying glass to examine my skin closely. She said this was to determine what sort of treatment I should have.

Then using the first in another series of creams, she massaged my face for about five minutes. Not all operators do this, but Theresa also massaged my shoulders, neck, and upper arms, down to the elbows. It was absolutely terrific. She wiped that cream off, covered my eyes with pads, turned on a little steam machine that used deionized water, and left the room. I was there for about ten minutes. I think the idea is to open your pores.

Then came the major event: cleansing the skin and pores. This operator was very good and used only her fingers to press around the pores to clean them. But I've had facials where a little instrument was used to apply pressure evenly around blackheads. If they open pimples, some places will use another instrument with an electric current to zap them and kill bacteria. Others use an antiseptic. After she was finished, Theresa used a toner or astringent.

Then she began the first of two masks. She told me the first would help nourish my skin; the second would seal the pores. Before putting on the masks, Theresa put cream around my eyes—they don't get a mask. She also put cream on my hands and elbows, covered my hands with baggies and tucked them into heated mittens. This is to soften your hands.

The first mask had aloe in it. The second had paraffin, and when she put it on, it got dry, but not hard. It made my skin unbelievably smooth.

Most facials last about an hour, but this one went on for a full hour and a half. Several people told me that they never saw my skin look so good.

The only problem—and this is typical—was that while she was putting on the masks, the operator started recommending products that she thought I should buy from the salon. I have a lot of facials, so I bought only a couple of small things—a seaweed mask for about $18 and some sunscreen, also about $18. The pressure to buy feels very intense because if you like your operator, you feel guilty when you don't buy.

Pat has a facial every month. When she was younger, she had very oily skin, and the advice at the time was that pores on oily skin always needed cleaning out. Pat got into the habit of having a facial once a month, and she continues this practice.

Typically, a facial in a large city will cost anywhere from $35 to $60, sometimes more, depending upon the type of masks that are used and the exclusiveness of the salon. Georgette Klinger, in New York, one of the largest and best-known salons, is currently charging $55 for one facial, and $195 for four of them.

The treatment is fairly standard: cleaning and one or more masks. The cleaning is more intensive for women with oily skin, and some salons advertise that their operators are specialists in noninstrumental cleaning.

Others swear by comedone extractors, little devices that apply pressure evenly around pimples and "pop" them out. The masks, which can be quite soothing, are made of a variety of ingredients, depending upon skin type. Most women say that they make their skin feel very smooth, but there is no hard evidence that indicates that these masks have any permanent effects.

The operators who give the facials are often European- or foreign-born, and many boast of a European training. They are usually also instructed to try to sell the product. It is customary to tip the operator. Most women tell me that they give 15 percent of the cost of the facial.

Mail Order

There are now several mail order companies that distribute catalogues that include skin care products. Most of these are moderately priced products sold at prices that are additionally reduced. The problem here is one of selection. If you have a specific product that you buy regularly, you may get a bargain.

Health Food Stores

And now a few words about natural cosmetics.

There are some ingredients that immediately spell out n-a-t-u-r-a-l to many people. These include vitamin E, aloe, jojoba oil, lecithin, almonds, honey, herbs, and plant extracts.

The customer for natural cosmetics is usually very concerned with questions of purity as well as safety. There is no reason why natural cosmetics should not be as safe as those prepared with synthetic ingredients, provided that there is adequate preservation within the formula. Botanicals spoil easily, something to keep in mind when mixing your own "kitchen cosmetics." Most reputable manufacturers of natural cosmetics are acutely aware of the problems of preservation. But here are some things to be aware of when buying "natural." If the product is touted as being completely natural, the preservative will probably be an antioxidant, such as vitamin A, E, or C. These are not as strong as the chemical preservatives, such as parabens (methyl or propyl), that are more often used in traditional cosmetics. The parabens extend the shelf life of the product. The antioxidants, wonderful as they are, will not be effective for more than six months to a year, top. Try to buy only products that are dated, and stay well within the limits. To prevent rancidity, I would also advise refrigeration for all natural creams and lotions.

I have nothing against the skin care products carried in the health food store; as a matter of fact, I once bought an apricot body lotion that smelled absolutely fabulous and was one of the best I've ever used. However, I don't live near such a store, and my shopping is therefore limited. But, from my reading of the various labels, I don't always see any major difference between the ingredients in regular cosmetics and those in natural cosmetics. This is particularly true when it comes to makeup and other color products.

If you buy a natural skin care product that you love, by all means keep using it. However, if you are shopping in a health food store to avoid preservatives or certain ingredients and are spending more to do this, I would check out the ingredients labels to see whether you are getting what you are paying for.

Some women also make the mistake of assuming that natural means that the product will be less irritating or have less potential as an allergen. This is not always the case.

Health food store employees rarely apply any pressure to buy; if anything, one sometimes gets the impression that the cosmetics and skin care shelf is the neglected stepchild.

Direct Selling and the Cosmetics Consumer

The first one to come calling was Avon. As a matter of fact, Avon started the whole business of selling door to door back in 1886, but they scored their biggest successes during the 1960s by using women to sell cosmetics to other women. Right now there are approximately 425,000 Avon representatives in the United States (over a million worldwide), and most of the sales are still made in the same way: The Avon representative takes your order, and delivers it a few days later, which is when you pay.

Back in the 1950s and early 1960s, women not only were happy with the product but enjoyed the extra social contact they derived from their relationship with the Avon representative. The women who worked for Avon, most of them housewives looking for some extra spending money, were equally satisfied.

But things began to change in the 1960s, as most of us remember. More and more women who wanted to get back into the workplace were getting chances to do just that. However, for companies like Avon (and Fuller Brush), it was never quite the same. Fewer women were home during the day, and fewer women were available for jobs as Avon representatives.

Then along came Mary Kay. Mary Kay Ash and her son Richard Rogers founded Mary Kay, and there is no question that Mary Kay herself has a real flair and made a big splash in the cosmetics world. In this case, it was a pink splash, because not only did Mary Kay live in a pink mansion and drive a pink car, she honored her strongest saleswomen with pink Cadillacs of their own. Mary Kay had a whole other way of direct selling cosmetics: the Party Plan. Here's how Party Plan works. The company representative approaches a woman, who has either been referred or who has attended another party, and this woman agrees to function as a "hostess" for a Mary Kay party and in turn invites a dozen or so of her nearest and dearest friends to her house for a Mary Kay party. She may provide coffee, tea, refreshments, etc. The company representative supplies the sales pitch and the demonstration. It's an easy way to get women to try something. They feel comfortable with their friends, but they also feel embarrassed if they don't buy something. These parties, which take place in the evening, don't interrupt the work life of a woman who works. In the early 1980s, Mary Kay doubled its sales; in 1982 their sales reached $36.6 million.

In the last few years, both Mary Kay and Avon have placed a great deal of emphasis on skin care products, and some of the sales methods have changed. In many cities, Avon has small outlets that one can walk into and order the product. You still have to wait a few days, but you still also pay on delivery.

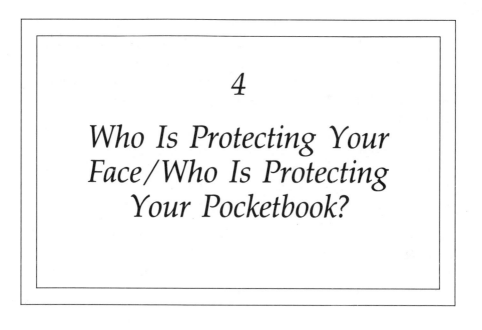

4

Who Is Protecting Your Face/Who Is Protecting Your Pocketbook?

I've discovered that the average woman doesn't have a clue about the ingredients included in the stuff she uses on her face. She is also blissfully unaware of whether or not any of these ingredients might be harmful, and she is similarly uneducated about any regulations that might exist to protect either her face or her pocketbook.

The regulations that protect the skin care consumer are limited, but such as they are, you should know about them. You should also be aware of the federal agencies that protect you not only from the potential of physical harm, but also from false and misleading advertising. Let's start with:

The FDA and the Food, Drug and Cosmetic Act

Until 1938, there was no Food, Drug and Cosmetic Act. Manufacturers, respectable and otherwise, could merchandise not only cosmetics, but also drugs, with little thought about consumer safety. Both suppliers and consumers were often frighteningly ignorant of the dangers that could be found in readily available products. Examples of the type of products that were sold in the late nineteenth century include a cough syrup that was laced with heroin and a popular baby syrup that used morphine to get the kid to snooze.

By the early twentieth century, a certain amount of blind trust had vanished, and more than a few Americans were becoming aware of the absence of standards in the manufacturing of food and drugs. Consequently, an agency that was known as the Bureau of Chemistry decided to test some food products then being sold. These tests resulted in the disclosure that there were products that contained harmful—or toxic—substances. This, in turn, resulted in the government's passing of the Pure Food and Drug Act of 1906. This act prohibited the interstate sale of adulterated or mislabeled food and drugs, but it was limited in scope and did nothing to protect the consumer from false therapeutic claims. It also provided no regulations that would make manufacturers test new drugs for safety. This omission ultimately resulted in a tragedy.

In 1937, a well-known company decided to include a new miracle drug, known as sulfanilamide, in a cough syrup. Unfortunately, they decided to combine the drug with an ingredient called diethylene glycol. Diethylene glycol is highly toxic, but because no tests were required to substantiate safety, it was put on the market without anyone realizing the potential for disaster. More than a hundred children died as a result of taking this cough syrup, and it became overwhelmingly apparent that new legislation was desperately needed.

However, when food and drug legislation was first considered, there were no provisions for the inclusion of cosmetics. After all, most people reasoned, what could be harmful in beauty preparations?

But in 1933 a serious cosmetics-related injury occurred, proving that cosmetics are not always benign substances. When using Lash Lure, a dark tint used in salons to color lashes and eyebrows, at least one young woman was blinded and others were injured by the coal tar dye that was an essential ingredient in the product. This injury prompted the regulations that expanded the proposed Food and Drug laws to include cosmetics. These were certainly not the first, or the last, injuries directly attributed to the use of a cosmetic product, but they contributed to a growing awareness of the need for laws governing the sale of cosmetics.

When the Food, Drug and Cosmetic Act of 1938 was passed, the FDA was given jurisdiction for enforcing its regulations. The laws, at least as far as cosmetics are concerned, are still much more limited than most people realize.

What the FDA Is Empowered to Do

Skin care products are viewed as cosmetics, and the primary law governing the composition of cosmetics is the Federal Food, Drug and Cosmetic Act. How cosmetics are labeled is governed by the Fair Packaging and Labeling Act. Both of these acts are enforced by the U.S. Food and Drug Administration, an agency of the Department of Health and Human Services. The FDA's activities include the following:

· consumer complaints and injury evaluations
· cosmetics registration activities
· chemical analysis and method development
· field inspections and compliance activities
· health hazard research
· regulation development
· public assistance and education

As you might imagine, because cosmetics generally present fewer potential risks than food or drugs, a relatively small portion of the agency's operating budget is set aside for cosmetics regulation. To give you some idea of how little, in the 1980s, when the agency's annual budget was approximately $321 million, the amount spent on cosmetics regulation came to about $2.5 million, which represents less than 1 percent of the total. The reality is that the FDA is severely limited by its budget in how far it can carry many of these activities. In an average year, for example, the FDA may make in the neighborhood of 400 on-site inspections of cosmetics manufacturers.

Cosmetics Labeling and Manufacturing Regulations

The regulations concerning cosmetics labeling were added to the Food, Drug and Cosmetic Act in 1977. Until then, when we bought a jar of cream or a blusher, we had no way of knowing what was included. This was terrific for the cosmetics industry. The secrecy not only helped manufacturers protect product formulas; it also helped them maintain the illusion that they were using ingredients far more glamorous than plain old petrolatum or mineral oil. Now when we shop, we can look at the label and know.

There is no confusion about the laws surrounding the labeling of cosmetic products; they are very specific. The outside container or wrapper of a cosmetic product must tell the consumer the manufacturer's name and the address of the manufacturer, packer, or distributor, the weight of the contents of the package, a list of the ingredients, and, when necessary, any cautionary or warning language. When listing the ingredients, the label should specify the following:

1. Ingredients present in the product in concentrations of more than 1 percent should be listed on the label in descending order of predominance. Ingredients present in concentrations of less than 1 percent may be grouped without regard to predominance.

I used to tell women that they could look at the first five ingredients listed and be able to identify the most important ones immediately. With skin care products, however, this is no longer true. Although the ingredients that are present in the heaviest concentrations will still be among the first five, many of the so-called magic or secret ingredients are present in very small quantities. An example of this is found in Estée Lauder's Night Repair, where sodium hyaluronate, a very important ingredient, is not among the first five listed.

2. Ingredients are supposed to be listed only by their recognized standard names.

If you're really interested in knowing more about this, check the *Cosmetic Ingredient Dictionary*, produced by the Washington-based Cosmetic, Toiletry and Fragrance Association, Inc. It provides a comprehensive source of approved nomenclature.

3. When a cosmetic also qualifies as a drug, the label for the product must list the drug ingredient(s) as "active ingredient(s)" at the top of the ingredients listing.

Many of us buy over-the-counter drugs regularly without being aware of the distinction that is made between them and cosmetics. Sunscreens are a good example of over-the-counter drugs, and if you pick up the sunscreen you use, you will be able to check out its active ingredients. Other examples include dandruff shampoos, acne medications, and hormone creams.

4. Specific fragrance ingredients do not have to be listed individually, and when a fragrance is present, it is sufficient for the manufacturer to note it on the label with one word—"fragrance"—without listing the specific ingredients from which the fragrance is derived.

I never could understand why manufacturers included fragrance in so many products since so many women complain of sensitivity to it. I

In A.M wash face w/facecloth rinced in tepid water, splash face ten to stimes, while damp apply moisturizer. (use La prairie skin conditioner $50 oz & complex is lotion $7. oz alternating the 2 creams) At night use soap (Lowila, pH balanced, by Westwood Labs in winter switch to Cetaphul Lotion.) Before Bed apply Capture skin care by Christian Dior $65 oz. Twice week exfoliate skin with Buf-Puf (gentle texture) for 30 seconds circular motion (it gets rid of dead skin cells & speeds up the process of cell renewal. Once a week polish skin w/oatmeal (pour some onto hand, wet it & scrub it around face. Rince carefully & apply moisturizer. Mask 1 egg + 1 T. honey + 1 T. cod Liver oil. Smear over face until dry. Rinse off w/tepid water. (This mask not for oily skin.) If skin gets greasy use a lohol free toner/astringent 2 to 3 times a week. (Lencome products = Tonique Douceur $8.75 for 5oz use 1 bottle tender a year). For Body hand lotion = Vaseline Intensive care. ① Use moisturizer at all times. ② Sunscreen for sun. (made by Westwood)

① Moisturizer by La Prairie Skin conditioner
- Complex 15 lotion
③) Lowite soap
, Cetaphil for winter (lotion)
③ Capture skin care (Christian Dior)
④ use Buf-Puf for exfoliation
⑤ Oatmeal to polish skin
⑥ mask 1 Egg   1 T. Honey 1 T. cod liver oil
⑦ Lancome = Hidrique Douceur
⑧ Vaseline Intensive care

discovered that fragrance is usually included to mask other chemical odors that might be considered unpleasant. In any event, the fragrance used in any one product can be made of a blend of many specific fragrances, in some cases, ten or more. It would be impossible for manufacturers to list them all.

5. If the FDA has accepted that a specific ingredient has trade-secret status, it does not have to be disclosed on the label. The ingredients are required, however, to be listed by the phrase "and other ingredients."

When I was working on my last book, I searched high and low to find some examples of products that included ingredients that had trade-secret status. I was able to find only one or two; this surprised me because I would have imagined from the advertising that many more of them were so-called secrets.

6. Color ingredients can be listed in any order, regardless of how much of the color is included in the product.

In skin care products, color is not as big a deal as it is in lip, eye, or foundation makeup. However, it is still found in several skin care lines; one is aware of it when the products are tinged yellow, green, pink, etc.

Warning Labels The FDA also requires appropriate warnings on three types of cosmetic products: feminine deodorant sprays, cosmetics packaged in aerosol containers, and cosmetics that have not been approved for safety by the manufacturers.

There is, for example, a regulation that says that *manufacturers* are supposed to substantiate the safety of their products before marketing. It says:

> Each ingredient used in a cosmetic product and each finished cosmetic product shall be adequately substantiated for safety prior to marketing. Any such ingredient or product whose safety is not adequately substantiated prior to marketing is misbranded unless it contains the following conspicuous statement on the principal display panel:
> "Warning—the safety of this product has not been determined."

Regulation Against "Poisonous or Deleterious Substances" There is a regulation against "adulterated" cosmetics, and the FDC Act provides that a cosmetic is deemed to be "adulterated . . . if it bears or contains any poisonous or deleterious substance which may render it injurious to users under the conditions of use prescribed in the labeling thereof, or, under such conditions of use as are customary or usual . . ."

The FDA may find a cosmetic adulterated if:

1. It is injurious to users under conditions of customary use because it contains, or its container is composed of, a potentially harmful substance.
2. It contains filth.
3. It contains a nonpermitted color additive.
4. It is manufactured or held under unsanitary conditions.

Prohibited Ingredients   There are very few prohibited or restricted ingredients. With few exceptions, a cosmetics manufacturer may use just about any raw material or combination of materials as ingredients in a product so long as they are not known to be harmful or injurious and market it without anyone's approval. Ingredients that are prohibited, or restricted, include: bithionol, mercury compounds, vinyl chloride, halogenated salicylanilides, zirconium complexes in aerosol cosmetics, chloroform, chlorofluorocarbon propellants, and hexachlorophene.

Hormone Ingredients   For a while there, some people expected hormone creams that contained estrogen to be marketed with greater enthusiasm, but it turned out that hormone creams create a problem. Estrogen can be absorbed through the skin, and women run the risk of absorbing enough estrogen to disrupt the menstrual cycle. Consequently, there is a regulation on the use of hormone creams. It reads: "The estrogen content of an over-the-counter product may not exceed 10,000 IU per ounce, and users must be directed to limit the amount of product applied daily so that no more than 20,000 IU of estrogen or equivalent be used per month."

Colors Permitted and Prohibited in Cosmetics   There are very strict rules concerning which colors can, and cannot, be included in cosmetic products. These regulations are most stringent when it comes to colors that can be used in the eye area. Many of the colors used in cosmetics are certified coal tar colors. Coal tar colors are prohibited for use around the eyes because they can cause serious injury and even blindness. One can recognize these colors by the initials D&C or FD&C preceding the color name and number. An example is D&C Yellow #10 or FD&C Yellow #6. Coal tar colors are prohibited from use in the eye area. The Code of Federal Regulation states:

> Section 135.01: The authorization contained in these regulations for the certification of coal tar colors shall not be considered to authorize the certification of any coal tar color for use in any article which is applied to the area of the eye. . . . The term "area of the eye" means the area enclosed within the circumference of the supra-orbital ridge and the infra-orbital ridge, including the eyebrow, the skin below the eyebrow, eyelids and eyelashes, the conjunctival sac of the eye, the eyeball, and the soft arcolar tissue that lies within the perimeter of the infra-orbital ridge.

In skin care products, coal tar colors would typically be considered an issue only in products that are used around the eyes, such as eye cream, or if a woman used her skin cream on her entire face, including around the eyes.

Steps the FDA Can Take to Enforce the FDC Act

If the FDA believes that a cosmetic product is either adulterated or incorrectly labeled, the FDA can send a notice of adverse findings or a regulatory letter, both of which are formal warnings, to the manufacturer.

A notice of adverse findings usually says that the agency believes that there has been some sort of violation or flaw, and the agency will request a reply within thirty days that will inform the agency of "each corrective step taken or intended to be taken including measures to prevent recurrence of the violation."

A regulatory letter is a more serious document. It pretty much signifies that the FDA is committed to start administrative or legal action "immediately if correction is not promptly achieved," and usually provides less time for response (often ten days).

An even more serious step for the FDA to take is a request that the manufacturer recall the product. The FDA regulations state: "A request from the Food and Drug Administration that a firm recall a product is reserved for urgent situations and is to be directed to the firm that has the primary responsibility for the manufacture and marketing of the product that is to be recalled."

A recall, which is usually voluntary, can begin when the firm discovers a problem with its product, or when the FDA finds the problem. It may involve the actual removal of products from the shelves, or it may be limited to a correction of the problem where it is located.

There are three classes of recalls, and the urgency with which the FDA deals with the products depends upon the type of recall that is involved.

A Class I recall is a situation in which there is reason to believe that use of, or exposure to, the product, will cause serious adverse health consequences, or even death.

A Class II recall is one in which the use of, or exposure to, the product, may cause temporary or medically reversible health problems, or where the probability of serious health consequences is remote.

A Class III recall is one in which the use of, or exposure to, a product is not likely to cause adverse health consequences.

Because I have always been curious about what sort of problems cause a recall, I got a list of recalls for some years in the early 1980s. When I took a quick look at products recalled during 1982 and 1983, for example, I saw an eyelash dye that included coal tar colors; an aloe moisturizing cream, which was found to be contaminated with bacteria; a batch of a very popular cream, which was manufactured (without the manufacturer's knowledge) with a nonpermitted color additive; a nail polish that was distributed without labeling; a shampoo that was found to be contaminated with bacteria; and a bubble bath that was prepared under unsanitary conditions.

A seizure, which is an action taken to remove a product from the marketplace because it is in violation of the law, is a more serious matter than a recall. The FDA initiates a seizure by filing a complaint with the U.S. District Court in the area in which the product is located. Then a U.S. marshall is called in to assume possession of the product until the matter is fully resolved.

There are many fewer seizures than recalls, and when it happens, the manufacturer usually has several problems, or at least one glaring one. In 1982 and 1983, products that were seized included a tanning tablet that contained a nonpermitted color additive; and a spray perfume that contained a prohibited propellant called chlorofluorocarbon.

Understanding the Difference Between a Drug and a Cosmetic

A drug *must undergo tests for safety and effectiveness before it is marketed.* A cosmetic *does not have to undergo tests for safety and effectiveness.*

Many consumers are confused about the different ways in which drugs and cosmetics are marketed and regulated. This is particularly true since some over-the-counter drugs, such as sunscreens, are also cosmetics. Another reason why consumers become confused is the heavy emphasis on scientific language in so many cosmetics ads. But it is important to remember that there is a difference between drugs and cosmetics, and there are many fewer regulations governing cosmetics.

The FDC Act defines cosmetics as "articles intended to be rubbed, poured, sprinkled, or sprayed on, or introduced into, or otherwise applied to the human body or any part thereof for cleansing, beautifying, promoting attractiveness, or altering the appearance, and articles intended for use as a component of any such articles; except that such term shall not include soap."

Most skin creams, lotions, clarifiers, eye creams, wrinkle creams, etc., easily fall under this definition.

Drugs are defined as "articles intended for use in the diagnosis, cure, mitigation, treatment or prevention of disease in man" and "articles (other than food) intended to affect the structure or any function of the body of man."

Any product that fits this definition, even when it provides a cosmetic function, is considered a drug, and, as such, it is required to undergo drug testing for both safety and effectiveness before being marketed.

Are Skin Care Products Safe?

We like to assume that skin care products have little potential for causing serious injuries, and despite a few notable exceptions, in which ingredients were used that later proved to be toxic, they have an enviable safety record. However, as more and different chemicals and chemical compounds find their way into skin care products, keep in mind that these products have not undergone the same type of rigid testing for safety as is required for new drugs, and, as any chemist is aware, any chemical can be toxic or dangerous under the right conditions or in sufficiently strong concentrations. In other words, nothing is absolutely safe.

Because skin care products contain many fewer coal tar colors, some of which have been questioned as potential carcinogens, they are probably safer than even most cosmetics. However, too often in the past, products and ingredients that were considered harmless have been proven otherwise. This is something that we should keep in mind as we read the advertisements for products that the manufacturers are claiming can have an effect on cell conditions.

With products that encourage cell renewal, for example, we should ask whether it is possible for there to be too much of a good thing. If cell renewal is accelerated beyond a certain point, the possibility of an inflammatory reaction exists, and this might produce problems. Also, we should bear in mind that not that much is yet known about what causes cells to divide, and there are conditions and illnesses in which it might not be wise to encourage such division.

Right now, approximately 8,000 chemicals are used in cosmetic products. In high enough concentrations, some of these chemicals are quite toxic. We simply don't know enough to say with absolute surety that none of the combinations used in skin care products have the potential for toxic effects.

Toxins can enter the body through the mucous membranes, by inhalation, by ingestion, or through skin absorption. When it comes to skin care products, insufficient information is available on just how real the possibility of skin absorption is. We know, for example, that mercury is highly toxic and accumulates in the body and we also know that mercury was once a permitted ingredient in cosmetic products. Whether or not there is anything now being used that has the same potential for toxicity as mercury is something we don't know. We can only hope that the modern skin care manufacturer is sufficiently knowledgeable and ethical, and that we, as skin care consumers, are not running any unnecessary risks. Because so few regulations exist on the use of cosmetics ingredients, we are dependent, more than some of us would like, on the ways in which the cosmetics industry regulates itself.

Self-Regulation and the Cosmetics Industry

Many people, when they refer to the cosmetics industry, use the term "self-regulated." What this means is that, in several very important areas, a policy has developed that allows the cosmetics industry to stand aside and serve as its own watchdog.

Among other things, this means that many of the regulations that do exist depend upon manufacturer cooperation, and frequently it is the cosmetics industry itself that is monitoring its own performance and safety standards.

This policy has come to be accepted practice for a few important reasons. The first, and not to be discounted, is the limited funds available to the Cosmetic Division of the Federal Drug and Food Administration. The second, and equally important, factor is the way in which the cosmetics industry has maneuvered and positioned itself as the primary proponent in the development of self-regulation. To understand this, we have to recognize the role of the Cosmetic, Toiletry and Fragrance Association. The CTFA is the powerful trade organization of the cosmetics industry. It represents approximately 250 companies, which, in turn, manufacture approximately 90 percent of all the cosmetic products marketed in the United States. It's fair to say that whenever a problem arises that affects the cosmetics industry, the CTFA, which was originally known as the Toilet Goods Association, is involved.

One of the basic laws of physics states that for every action, there is an opposite and equal reaction. When Ralph Nader and other committed consumerists began to delve into the quality and safety of various industries, these industries often responded in kind. As consumerism grew, so the CTFA became more efficient and organized in attempting to prevent government regulations from controlling the development of the cosmetics industry.

The regulatory environment in the United States goes through many changes, more often than not depending upon the political administration in power. With some administrations, it is more stringent; other times, it is less restrictive. During the Reagan years, there was an emphasis on government deregulation. During the early 1970s, when consumerism flourished, there was a sense that more regulations were required, and several attempts were made to enlarge the activities of the FDA as well as to broaden the scope of the FDC Act.

The basic controversy arose then because there were consumer groups who believed that the FDA should oversee cosmetics almost as diligently as they did drugs and, hence, "clear" cosmetics before they were marketed. A bill was introduced that spoke to this issue and that also called for the following:

· mandatory FDA registration of cosmetic products
· submission of all cosmetics formulas to the FDA
· required reporting to the FDA on adverse reactions.

The cosmetics industry obviously did not want this much regulation, and it served its best interests to do whatever was necessary to prevent the passage of such a bill.

Rather than run the risk of any further attempts at legislation, the CTFA, acting as spokesperson for the cosmetics industry, filed a petition that asked that the FDA adopt a different program. This is now the one that is used. It calls for voluntary registration of cosmetics companies with the FDA, voluntary filing of product information, and voluntary disclosure of adverse reactions and consumer complaints.

This is what this means:

· Registration of manufacturing and packing establishments.

Although the FDC Act does not require cosmetics firms to register with the FDA, the FDA encourages manufacturers to do so. When a firm registers voluntarily, it is issued a registration number, but this does not indicate that the FDA has approved the firm or any of its products. Currently, almost half of all cosmetics manufacturers are registered with the FDA; this number, which includes almost all the major companies, comes to close to a thousand.

· Registration of cosmetics ingredients, raw materials, and product formulations.

The response to the voluntary registration of ingredients and product formulations is nowhere near as enthusiastic; there are nearly 8,000 cosmetics ingredients, and fewer than 4,000 are registered; approximately 20,000 product formulations are registered.

· Voluntary reporting of cosmetic product experiences.

This includes information that the company receives concerning adverse reactions; fewer than 100 companies are now participating.

The CTFA and the Cosmetic Ingredient Review

Much of the testing of cosmetics ingredients for safety is done by the Cosmetic Ingredient Review, which was established by the CTFA. For example, it sponsored the major testing on the colors that were included in cosmetics and that were suspected of being carcinogenic.

Long-range testing for safety is a very expensive process. With its current budget, the FDA cannot afford to do it. The CTFA, in its role as representative of the largest cosmetics manufacturers, is probably the major group able to assume responsibility for such testing. However, the fact remains that CTFA is an industry-funded organization. It is not responsible to any consumer group and it is not a government organization. By definition, it owes its allegiance to the people who support it. That being so, one can't help questioning the CTFA's objectivity.

The NAD, Advertising Self-Regulation, and Skin Care Ads

Many consumers who are concerned about truth in advertising might be interested in knowing that the advertising community also has a system of self-regulation. It is known as NAD, the National Advertising Division Council of Better Business Bureaus, and the NARB, the National Advertising Review Board. This system of self-regulation was established in 1971 by the American Advertising Federation, the American Association of Advertising Agencies, the Association of National Advertisers, and the Council of Better Business Bureaus to help maintain standards of truth and accuracy in national advertising.

NAD collects and evaluates data to see whether advertisers' claims can be substantiated. If it finds the substantiation is insufficient or unsatisfactory, the advertiser is asked to modify or discontinue the ad. It chooses its cases by monitoring national advertisements and by responding to consumer complaints. In several instances, NAD has investigated advertisements for skin care products.

One case, for example, involved the advertisements that were done for Elizabeth Arden's Millennium. In that instance, they found the claims that Arden made for the advertised product were substantiated.

Another case involved an early ad for Estée Lauder's Night Repair that stated, "Use it tonight and wake up to better looking skin." When NAD reviewed the advertisements and the material dealing with Night Repair's effects, they questioned whether the data would substantiate the claim of such dramatic improvements in one night. Lauder then agreed to clarify in the advertisements that improvements are most apparent with regular, nightly use.

The Federal Trade Commission and the Role It Assumes in Cosmetics Marketing

The other federal agency that directly affects the way in which cosmetics are marketed is the Federal Trade Commission, or FTC. The FTC, established in 1914, is directly concerned with monitoring and regulating the marketing practices, including advertising, used in the sale of all consumer products, including cosmetics, as well as food, drugs, and other health care products.

It is sometimes difficult to understand where the FDA's mandate leaves off and where the FTC's begins. The FDA is in charge of labeling cosmetic products, including everything written on the label and all the *promotional literature* in the package. The FTC is in charge of what is said or written in all *advertising* in all media, including radio, television, and magazines.

The FTC is an independent federal agency with five commissioners and a staff of more than 1,000 employees who are located in Washington as well as in regional offices.

The staff of the FTC is responsible for enforcing the regulations contained within the Federal Trade Commission Act; this act expressly prohibits "unfair methods of competition in or affecting commerce," and "unfair or deceptive acts or practices in or affecting commerce."

In addition, the FTC Act prohibits false advertising for food, drugs, devices, and cosmetics. When the FTC Act refers to advertising, it clearly *means* advertising; it does *not* mean promotional material included in packaging. If you see it on television, read it in a magazine or book, hear it on the radio, and it is paid for, it is considered advertising. Promotional material included in the package is considered labeling, and the FDA, not the FTC, has jurisdiction.

In the FTC Act, false advertisement is defined to mean advertising that is misleading. When deciding what is misleading, the FTC commissioners are supposed to consider not only what is said, but also what is not said, or implied, and what should be stated in an advertisement in order for it to be clear.

An advertisement, for example, is considered false if it does not tell, or reveal, to the consumer facts that are important in light of representations in the advertisement. It is also considered false if it fails to reveal facts concerning any possible negative consequences that could result from customary and usual use of the product.

When Pure Puffery Needs Verification— Unfair Competition

The FTC, not the FDA, is also empowered to regulate unfair competition, and this includes false advertising. FTC policy is that advertisers have to substantiate claims before they are made.

The FTC has traditionally maintained a very low profile as far as the skin industry is concerned. They have, for example, been much more involved in food advertising; you may remember that television networks began some year ago to ask their advertisers to prove claims made in commercials.

Since truth in advertising extends to photographs, advertisers were no longer allowed to doctor their products to make them more attractive when photographed and thus create distortions in what the consumer sees. Soup manufacturers, for instance, could not make the vegetables float to the surface by adding marbles to the bottom of the bowl. With many advertisements, such as those for food or cars or fur coats, the restrictions are fairly clear.

Using Consumer Preference Data to Substantiate Claims But when it comes to skin care and cosmetics in general, it is very difficult to distinguish between pure puffery and claims that need verification. By and large, if a company says, for example, "Our night cream, Lady Macbeth's Hand Creme Deluxe, makes your fingers feel real fabulous," they don't have to prove a thing.

However, if they claim that Lady Macbeth's Hand Creme Deluxe does more for your skin than any other hand cream on the market, they have to prove it. There is no objective way to prove that statement, but there is a way to support it and thus attempt substantiation. The traditional way is an old standby called consumer preference testing. What this means, essentially, is that somebody goes out and does a survey, or has a panel of consumers evaluate a product or compare several products. The data attained have to be specific and clear before they can be used to promote the product.

If they are not, a competitor may well take issue with your statement. For example: A large, well-known, established, and prestigious company promoted a new shampoo that featured a beautiful adult model. She issued the following statement: ". . . in shampoo tests with over 900 women like me, [my shampoo] got higher ratings than Prell for body, higher than Flex for conditioning, and higher than Sassoon for strong, healthy looking hair."

Sassoon stated that they felt the ad was false and they filed suit. The court found that the original shampoo manufacturer had not done the kind of testing that would give them the right to make these claims. They had not given the 900 women the sort of test in which they judged the products tried against each other. Instead, some of the women tried the original shampoo, some tried Prell, some tried Flex, and some tried Sassoon. Then they were asked to rate each product, and the ratings were compared against each other. The court held that since these were not blind paired tests in which each of the women could compare the products but blind single testings, there were insufficient data to support the claim in the ads. The court also found that the ad was misrepresentative when the model claimed "900 women like me" because many of the respondents were not sophisticated adult women but teenage girls aged 13–18.

In this case, it was apparent that the original manufacturer was not trying to mislead. What had happened was that they had originally planned the test, not so they would have material for advertising, but just to get market research data on how women responded to their new product. Then someone decided, since they had such good results, that it might make sense to make better use of the research material. Voilà, the model's claim.

The thing to keep in mind with consumer data is that it is sufficient substantiation for a manufacturer to claim that his product can make skin feel good, but it is not enough to make a more scientific claim. If a manufacturer wants to say that a specific product cures a specific condition, clinical tests are required, and if someone wants to market the product as a drug, the product must undergo the sort of testing used for new drugs.

Subjective Evaluation—The Human Element A   major   stumbling block—both for manufacturers who are trying to prove a claim and for consumers who are trying to understand the language of a claim—is that there are few objective methods available to evaluate improvement or changes in a skin's condition.

One case involves two large companies, which manufacture skin care aimed at the average consumer; it is indicative of some of the problems involved. Litigation arose between Chesebrough-Pond's, who manufacture Vaseline Intensive Care Lotion, and Procter & Gamble, whose competing product is Wondra. Vaseline Intensive Care said in its promotion, ". . . when it comes to relieving dry skin, no leading lotion beats Vaseline Intensive Care Lotion," and Wondra's copy said ". . . relieves dry skin better than the leading lotion."

Obviously those were fighting words, and each side backed its right to claim greater effectiveness in dealing with dry skin with clinical tests, while trying to prove that the competing product was inferior and the tests supplied for the competing product were insufficient. To do this, a company might say that the study used the wrong samples, analyzed data incorrectly, etc.

The court responded by basically saying, "Who knows?" The opinion read in part:

> Neither of the parties has proven successfully that the other has chosen tests and conducted them in a manner to mislead the public. Courts are not always able to determine whether an advertising claim is true or false . . . we are dealing with rough tests that have no certifiable standards and that rest upon nothing more than subjective evaluations of skin conditions. . . . The parties are sparring to obtain commercial advantage over what is at most a cosmetological distinction.

This inability to decide on cosmetological distinction is what makes it so difficult to get a truly unbiased opinion on the effectiveness of most skin care products.

Truth in Advertising and How Its Meaning Has Changed

In recent years, the FTC has assumed a very laid-back attitude as far as cosmetics and skin care advertising is concerned. They seem to have taken the position that the individual consumer's response is subjective, and that the consumer is capable of deciding for herself whether or not the product truly works as claimed. If it doesn't, obviously she does not have to buy the product another time, and since the only directly assessable damage is limited to the cost of the product, a full-scale effort against cosmetics claims does not seem warranted. A jar of cold cream does not, after all, cost as much as a new luxury automobile, when a questionable advertising claim would elicit a much greater response.

This was not always the case. In 1944, there was a fascinating case concerning a product called Rejuvenescence Cream. In that case, the court found that advertising for the product falsely represented that the cream would restore the appearance of youth to the skin. In the light of today's inflated skin care claims, the court's decision, then, is so interesting that I'm quoting part of it:

> . . . while the wise and worldly may well realize the falsity of any representations that the present product can roll back the years, there remains "that vast multitude" of others who, like Ponce de León, still seek

the fountain of youth. . . . The average woman, conditioned by talk or magazines and over the radio of vitamins, hormones, and God knows what, might take rejuvenescence to mean that this is one of the modern miracles and is something which would actually cause her youth to be restored. . . . It is for this reason that the commission may insist upon the most literal truthfulness in advertisements . . . and should have the discretion, undisturbed by the courts, to insist, if it chooses, upon a form of advertising clear enough so that, in the words of the prophet Isaiah, "wayfaring men, though fools, shall not err therein."

You can see by this decision that the courts in 1944 were much more protective of the female consumer; they were also significantly more condescending. It would have been better perhaps if they could have maintained an attitude of protection toward the consumer without giving it a sexist bias.

It is interesting to note that the last time a serious case concerning consumer claims came up was in the 1960s. In this instance, there were several products, including one from Coty known as Line Away and another from Hazel Bishop called Sudden Change, that were the subject of an FDA action. Both of these products were temporary wrinkle removers. The formula included a bovine serum albumin that, when dried, formed a film over wrinkles, thus making the wrinkles less obvious.

In these cases, under the Food, Drug, and Cosmetic Act the courts have explained that medical-type product claims should be looked at and interpreted from the perspective of a very impressionable consumer. The courts have reasoned that if "ignorant, unthinking, or credulous" consumers could be misled into believing that these products were genuine wrinkle removal drugs, then they were incorrectly promoted and labeled as merely cosmetics. Once a cosmetic is deemed a drug, it must be reviewed and cleared by the FDA.

It would be unrealistic, as well as ill-founded, for anyone today to consider the female consumer as particularly credulous or unthinking. However, no one expects major manufacturers of reputable skin care products to purposely mislead, misdirect, or misinform the skin care consumer, who is stereotypically, but nonetheless probably accurately, portrayed as being a woman.

If the stereotypical male purchaser of four-wheel-drive vehicles was being misinformed in car ads, no one would accuse him of extremes of credulity. Instead, people would point a finger at the advertiser. I think it's fair to say that the average skin care consumer expects and deserves the same degree of federal protection, as well as respect.

TWO

Becoming Your Own Beauty Expert

5

What You Need to Know About Your Skin

If we decide to buy a car, used or new, we don't put blind faith in the car salesman, but try to get more information. We talk to friends, we visit the local mechanic, and we call up our cousin Joe who really *knows* about cars. We visit different showrooms and car lots, we investigate ads in the paper, and sometimes we read leading consumer-oriented publications. Eventually we get enough information to make a reasonable, and informed, decision. But still we often take the car on trial and have a mechanic look at it first.

When it comes to the skin on our faces, however, we have many fewer "experts" we can trust. The "expert" at the beauty counter is primarily interested in selling the product. Most dermatologists don't have the time to investigate skin care products, and even if we found one who did, we could hardly go running in every time we wanted to buy a new cleansing product.

I am absolutely convinced that the only way the female skin care consumer can take care of her skin and make informed choices is to become her own beauty expert.

Knowing your individual skin type is the first step in having terrific skin. The second step is knowing how to manage and protect it. But what do you want to protect it from? Many of the women I speak to have only one answer to that question. They say they want to protect it from the ravages of time; they want their skin to stay young looking as long as possible. But wrinkles are not the only things that can detract from your good looks. Other not so wonderful things can happen to your face. If you made a list of all the everyday skin problems that you want to avoid, the list would look something like this:

· blemishes
· pimples
· whiteheads
· acne and other oily skin flare-ups
· acne scarring
· scaling, flaking dry skin
· premature aging
· chapping, chafing
· exaggerated lines and wrinkles
· pigment changes and uneven tone
· brownspots
· sagging
· large pores
· sun damage
· sensitive skin

This is rather a long list, but most of these skin problems can be prevented. Sun protection will prevent photoaging, including premature sagging and exaggerated lines. Moisturizing with the correct ingredients will help alleviate many of the signs of dry skin. Proper evaluation and treatment of acne should prevent most scarring, and avoiding the wrong cosmetic products can help prevent further flare-ups. Concerned about pigment changes? Again, prevention is the name of the game. Prevention is also important when it comes to so-called sensitive skin. Many dermatologists now believe that women who have done too much for their skin are most likely to end up with facial skin that is easily irritated. Simple dry skin, of course, is inexpensively alleviated. Unfortunately, you can't do anything permanent about large pores, but you can make them appear smaller, at least temporarily.

The problem is that to accomplish all this preventive care, you need to know:

· what products to buy and how to use them
· what products not to buy and why

Knowing what to buy depends upon knowing more about skin in general, so that you can understand the language in skin care ads and promotions in order to determine what's real and what's not, and your skin type, so that you can manage it and choose the appropriate products.

Protecting Your Skin—Rule 1: Learn More About Skin and How It Functions

I want to try Retin-A, but someone told me that once I use it I can never again go in the sun. I don't know what that means, and I'm not sure if it is worth it.

I recently bought a moisturizer because the salesperson said it would "penetrate the epidermis" and help fight "free radical damage." Afterward, I realized that I didn't know what she was talking about. What was she talking about?

I have very oily skin, but I don't usually have pimples, except when I try to use makeup. Then I break out like crazy. This has also happened a couple of times when I bought some cleansing products thinking they would help get rid of the oil. Why does that happen?

Many of the ads for skin care products talk about increasing cell renewal. What does that mean, and why does this make your skin look younger?

These questions all point up one fact: The only way you can make informed choices about skin care products as well as dermatological procedures and treatments is to learn something about your skin. Facts about your skin may be basically boring, but knowing them can ultimately save you time, money, and aggravation. Most of the stuff that's written about skin starts off by telling the female reader that skin is the largest organ of her body. Then it goes on to tell her how many yards of it she has draped around her, sort of like flowered chintz.

To be perfectly honest, I wish I didn't have to rehash all the usual information about the skin and its layers, etc. However, if you buy face cream, you have been bombarded with advertisements and promotional material that emphasizes the new, "scientific" approach to marketing contemporary products. Unless you understand the "science" part of the ads, how can you be sure of exactly what the company is claiming? Or, just as important, whether it is something that you want, or need. So, here goes.

When you look at your hands, all you see is one continuous flesh-colored sheet of cellular tissue that you call skin. But if you had high-powered equipment, you would be able to see that it is really many sheets of tissue made up of many independent cells. These sheets and cells have different functions.

The skin has two separate and distinct segments or units. The outermost segment is called the epidermis. The segment beneath it is known as the dermis. These two units, the dermis and the epidermis, meet at a junction called the basement membrane.

The Epidermal Layer

The cells of the epidermis are stratified into sheets as follows:

The top layer of the epidermis, which itself has fifteen to twenty cellular layers, is known as the stratum corneum, or horny layer.

The next layer down is called the stratum granulosum.

Beneath that is the stratum spinosum.

At the bottom of the epidermis is the basal layer or germinative layer.

The Cells of the Epidermis The epidermis, which is the segment of skin that you see, is made up of several layers of epidermal cells; it is thinnest on the eyelids and thickest on the palms of your hands and soles of your feet.

The epidermis acts as the body's first layer of defense against the environment and serves to impede the entrance of micro-organisms, ultraviolet radiation, and toxic substances. The epidermis, which has no blood vessels or nerves, is, of course, made up of more cells than you and I can count. There are different types of epidermal cells. Following are the most important ones.

· *Keratinocytes* make up close to 80 percent of all epidermal cells. They are responsible for performing and maintaining the skin's barrier function. They got this name because they are made of keratin, which is a protein high in sulfur. There are two forms of keratin: hard keratin, found in hair and nails; and soft keratin, found in epidermal cells.

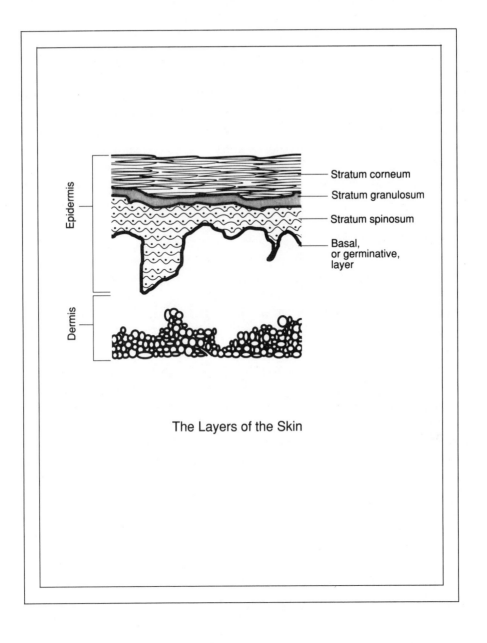

Epidermis

Dermis

Stratum corneum

Stratum granulosum

Stratum spinosum

Basal,
or germinative,
layer

The Layers of the Skin

- *Melanocytes* synthesize melanin. The amount of melanin in our skin is the primary determinant of skin color. The darker you are, the more melanin you have. Melanin in the epidermis is also what protects us from ultraviolet light. The more melanin-rich your skin is, the less vulnerable you are to ultraviolet light.
- *Langerhans cells* make up only 3 to 4 percent of all epidermal cells, but they are extremely important because of the role they play in the body's immune responses. Because the epidermis is the body's first line of defense against outside infectious agents, it is believed that the Langerhans cell may play a vital role in protecting the skin from outside invaders.

Cell Renewal: Getting Rid of Old Skin Cells Encourages New Skin Cells

When skin care ads talk about helping your skin look younger, regenerating skin cells, or plumping up your skin cells, they are talking about the cells in your epidermis. You are familiar with those products that claim to accelerate cell renewal. The cells they are renewing are in the epidermis.

As long as you are alive and breathing, your epidermal cells are in a continous state of regeneration and renewal. The only thing that changes as you age is how long it takes for new cells to form and find their way to the surface.

New epidermal cells are formed at the basal layer, the bottom layer of the epidermis. When they are first formed, they are round and "plump." These cells travel through the four epidermal layers until they reach the surface or top layer, the stratum corneum. As they travel, they get older and flatter looking, and by the time they reach the stratum corneum, the layer of skin that people see when they look at you, they are very flat indeed, and are ready to be shed or scraped off. This process of shedding is called desquamation.

When you use a Buf-Puf on your face, or a scrub of any kind, or even a washcloth, you are accelerating the process of desquamation. All that means is that you are scraping off dead, old skin cells. Many of the beauty articles that are written also refer to this process as exfoliation.

In dermatological language, the time it takes for the new cells that are formed in the bottom layer (basal layer) of the epidermis to travel through the various layers until they reach the top layer (stratum corneum) is known as transit time. Cell turnover is the phrase that is used when we are talking about how long it takes cells to replace themselves.

As we get older, cell turnover time slows down. When a woman is twenty, the cells in the top layers of the epidermis will be sloughed off and replaced every two or three weeks. When that same woman is eighty, the replacement can take up to twice as long.

If the cells take longer to reach the surface, they are necessarily older by the time they get there. Since the older skin cell is dryer and flatter, the next question is: Does the fact that the individual cells are actually older contribute to the look of aging skin, and, if that is the case, will the skin look younger—even on a mature woman—if the turnover or cell renewal time is speeded up?

Since the epidermis is in a continuous state of self-replacement or turnover, with new cells being born in the basal layer to replace the old cells being shed from the stratum corneum, it follows that if we speed up the rate at which the cells in the stratum corneum are being desquamated or shed, we will speed up the rate at which new cells are formed to replace them.

The cosmetic means by which cell renewal can be speeded up include:

· Using a mild irritant on the skin, which will induce more rapid desquamation.

Many dermatologists have pointed out to me that the reason why some skin care products make a claim of cell renewal is that they include an ingredient that induces a mild irritation that in turn speeds up the process of cell renewal.

· Using a mild abrasive such as a scrub or cleansing grains, both of which will also induce more rapid desquamation.

It is hoped that this acceleration process will make the skin look younger because the cells in the stratum corneum will always be "newer" ones that will therefore be able to retain moisture more effectively and, hence, have the plump look of younger cells. Incidentally, dermatologists also speed up this process of cell renewal whenever they use an "acid peel" on the face such as retinoic acid; dermabrasion, which is a mechanical process, is another medical procedure that revs up epidermal cell renewal.

A Plump Epidermal Cell Looks Younger Than a Dry One

A lot of the ads I've read talk about a product giving the cells a "plump" look. They indicate that that will make the skin look younger. What actually makes a skin cell look plump?

The more moisture (water) a skin cell retains, the plumper and more filled-out it looks. Several women have asked me about the ad language that talks about "plumper"-looking cells. What the ads are talking about are the cells of the stratum corneum layer of the epidermis. Therefore, the question is asked: Can we introduce moisture into the stratum corneum, causing the cells and skin to look younger and plumper?

And the answer would have to be yes. The stratum corneum can absorb, and with some help retain, moisture, and there is no question about it—skin that is moist and well hydrated looks younger than skin that is dry and dehydrated. And that's what most moisturizing products are all about.

Hiding Below the Epidermis—You and Your Dermis

Most of your skin, even though you don't see it, is dermis. The dermis, which protects your body from injury and stores water, is what gives your skin its strength. The dermis also determines major skin features, such as wrinkles and thickness.

People often say that the skin never forgets. What they really should say is that the dermis never forgets. When epidermal cells age and are sloughed off every few weeks, you get a brand new epidermis, but you always have the same old dermis. It is the dermis that maintains the skin's memory. If you have a scar, for example, it involves the dermis because damage to the dermis results in the production of fibroblasts, or cells that produce collagen fibers. A scar has its base in the dermis and is a combination of fibroblast cells and collagen fibers, which do not duplicate themselves in the way that epidermal cells do.

When you buy skin care products, you hear a lot about collagen. Collagen is the primary component of the dermis. It is a fibrous protein and the major connective tissue of the skin. We also hear a lot about elastin, another fibrous connective tissue that is found in the dermis.

There are other connective tissues of a nonfibrous variety found in the dermis. They form a substance that is sometimes called the ground substance. This ground substance has a terrific capacity to absorb and hold moisture, and it is made up of glycosaminoglycans or mucopolysaccharides, words that we have all seen in skin care ads or articles. These include chondroitin sulfate, dermatan sulfate, and hyaluronic acid. If you read the ingredients labels on skin care products, you have probably noticed hyaluronic acid in several Estée Lauder products as well as products in the Shiseido line.

More About the Collagen and Elastin in Your Dermis It sometimes seems as though collagen is included as an ingredient in almost all skin care lines. The collagen that is included in face creams and moisturizers comes from animal skin, usually calves'.

Within your dermis, collagen is found in bundles of tiny little fibers. When a scientist looks at collagen through a microscope, what is seen might be compared to a closely knit piece of wicker work.

Like collagen, elastin is also found in small bundles, but the two types of tissue are not normally together in the same bundle. Instead, they are found next to each other. Collagen, which comprises more than 70 percent of the dermis, is the predominant type of fiber bundle, and it is bordered by the bundles of elastin.

When you smile, grimace, or frown, elastin, which is the major component of the elastic fibers that are necessary to bring the skin back to its normal shape, has a role to play.

If you use a skin care product that includes collagen, do not make the mistake of assuming that this automatically means that you will be bolstering your skin's natural collagen supply. The collagen molecule cannot penetrate your skin because it is much too large to be absorbed by the epidermis. However, collagen is a very valuable skin care ingredient because it is such an effective moisturizing agent. However, it does not follow that applying collagen on the surface of your skin means that it is going to make its way through the layers of skin down to the dermis and increase your skin's natural supply of collagen.

Also, you should be aware that there are different types of collagen, and the skin experts number them—Collagen I, Collagen IV, etc.

Elastin is included in some skin care products, but nowhere near as much as collagen. It, too, cannot be absorbed by the epidermis.

The Basement Membrane or Dermal/Epidermal Junction

Lately I have begun to see the term "basement membrane" in articles concerning skin, and the impression I get from people I talk to is that more emphasis is going to be placed on the role it plays. The basement membrane is a connecting membrane located between the epidermis and the dermis, and experts tell me that it serves several important functions in relaying communications between the dermis and the epidermis. It also plays a role in supplying nutrients from blood vessels located in the dermis to the epidermis. Like the dermis, the primary component of the basement layer is collagen, but it is a different type of collagen.

Within Your Skin

Blood Supply Within your dermis are located the vessels that carry blood and oxygen to your skin. As you know, when your circulation is stimulated, your skin turns rosy or red. When circulation is poor, skin color reflects it with pallor. Typically, skin circulation slows down as we get older. That's one of the reasons why your face gets paler as you age.

Some of the skin care ads have referred to "improved microcirculation." When you see this type of claim, what it usually means is that something is being applied to the skin that brings blood up to the epidermis. Witch hazel is an old-fashioned ingredient that is perhaps best known in this regard.

Lymph System Your lymph vessels provide a drainage system that removes waste.

Nerves Touch, pain, heat, cold, itch, etc.—all of these messages of comfort and discomfort are conveyed by the nerves contained within the dermis.

Sweat Glands The sweat glands that keep us comfortable in the summer are also found within the dermis. There are two different kinds of sweat glands, the apocrine and the eccrine. Apocrine glands are connected to hair follicles and are found under the arm, in the genital area, and in the nipples. The secretion from the apocrine glands is released into sebaceous follicles.

Eccrine glands, which are found all over the body, have their own ducts and pores for the release of sweat. Their role is vital to the regulation of body temperature.

Sebaceous Glands The sebaceous glands, which secrete lipids, including sebum, are implicated in oily skin and acne (heavy sebum production) and dry skin (low sebum production). They are found in all areas of the skin with the exception of the palms of the hands and the soles of the feet. The oil that these glands secrete has a great deal to do with the way your skin looks. Ideally, the sebaceous glands secrete just enough oil to give it a smooth shield that softens the skin and keeps moisture locked in. With too much oil, you run the risk of clogged pores, blackheads, and whiteheads. With too little, the skin dries out and fine lines begin forming.

Hair Follicles Although hair serves no vital function in our lives, we are deeply distressed when it grows in an abnormal fashion. If we have too little hair, we are distraught. On the other hand, some women always seem to be battling the appearance of too much hair in places such as the face, legs, or arms. Hair, which is also made up of keratin, gets its color from pigment contained in melanocytes. When pigment lessens with age, the hair becomes gray or white.

For whatever it's worth, hair tends to turn gray on different parts of the body at different ages. Beard hair is usually the first to gray; scalp hair begins the graying process around the temples. Most Caucasians begin to gray between the ages of thirty and fifty. In general, blacks don't start to gray until later in life.

Underneath the Skin—The Subcutaneous Layer

If you could peek underneath your dermis, you would discover a layer of subcutaneous fat. This layer, which keeps you from being nothing but skin and bones, is sometimes called the hypodermis, and it insulates the body and actually protects your skin from coming into direct contact with your bones.

What Happens to Aging Skin

When skin care companies address themselves to products that will help the consumer look younger, they take into consideration all the changes that take place as skin ages. When it comes to aging and skin, the first thing to remember is that there are two separate and distinct forms of skin aging.

1. *True aging.* This is the kind you can't do much about. It happens to everyone.

   A great deal of time, money, and energy have been devoted to trying to find out why aging takes place, but so far there are no easy answers. When it comes to skin, all we basically have are descriptions.

2. *Photoaging.* This is the kind that is brought on by sun damage, and there is a great deal that can be done to prevent it.

   The fact is that many of the more dramatic, and negative, changes that we see in the skin, and that we associate with aging, are not necessary. They are the result of photoaging and they can be avoided.

When dermatologists examine aging skin, they notice several striking changes. Some of these changes also concern cosmetic scientists in their search for products that address the issues involved in aging skin.

- As skin ages, there is a flattening of the dermal/epidermal junction or basement layer and a reduction in the adhesion formed between the dermis and epidermis. This pulling away of the two layers of the skin probably means that there is less transference of information between the cells as well as a diminishment in efficiency of nutrient transfer.
- As skin ages, there is a decrease in the rate at which epidermal cells replace themselves. It is estimated that a decrease of about 30 to 50 percent takes place between the ages of thirty and eighty.
- As skin ages, its ability to heal and repair itself declines.
- As skin ages, there is a reduction in the number of melanocytes, and the skin's ability to protect against ultraviolet radiation is reduced.
- Langerhans cells are significantly reduced, and this reduction is associated with a lowering of immune response in the elderly.
- The dermis become thinner, and there is a reduction in certain types of dermal cells.
- Elastin fibers in the dermis are altered and become thicker.
- Enzymes necessary for collagen stabilization begin to decline.
- There is a decrease in certain mucopolysaccharides, particularly hyaluronic acid, which bind water to the skin.
- Blood vessels in the skin decrease and circulation decreases.
- Sebum production decreases.
- Sweat production decreases.
- Vitamin D production decreases.
- Soluble collagen decreases and insoluble collagen increases.

You don't need a medical degree to realize that the skin of an eighty-year-old looks different from that of a sixty-year-old and substantially different from that of a twenty-year-old. When you use your fingers to pinch up a piece of skin from a mature person, it takes longer to bounce back to its normal shape than if you were doing the same thing with young skin. But it is much harder to pinpoint exactly where and how these changes take place. We know that many of the more pronounced wrinkles and premature aging are caused by sun damage, but the sun is not responsible for all the age-related changes in the skin. Why do hormones and sebum levels change? Why and how do collagen and elastin change? What causes the loss of elasticity and strength?

These are all questions that researchers ask, but they don't have any answers or solutions. For the moment, all that can be done is to describe some of what occurs when skin ages and then try to resolve that issue. We know that aging skin is dry, for example, so we try to replace moisture in the hope that it will look younger.

Protecting Your Skin—Rule 2: Understand Your Skin and What Makes It Special

Before you say that you know your skin type, and skip to the next chapter, let me tell you that the odds are in favor of your being wrong in your assessment. Knowing your skin type is the most important element in choosing appropriate cosmetic and skin care products. I'm not alone in stressing this; rafts of magazine articles and books have talked about it, the cosmetics salespeople talk about it, and most companies manufacture products specified for oily, dry, or normal skin. Despite this, when Dr. James Leyden, a professor of dermatology at the University of Pennsylvania, recently asked a group of consumers to assess their skin type, he discovered that most were wrong. The likelihood is that you, too, don't know your own skin type. I think this happens for several reasons:

1. You may have been misinformed by a cosmetics salesperson.

Some cosmetics salespeople have been well trained and are really uncanny in determining skin type. Others are amazingly inept. The cosmetics salesperson is often at a real disadvantage in determining skin type. When you are in a store, there is a good possibility that you are wearing moisturizer or foundation, and your skin may appear oilier than it truly is. Or you may be using a drying soap and are wearing no moisturizer, and your skin appears drier than it really is.

Visual analysis, which is all a salesperson can do, is best done on clean skin that has been left alone for at least thirty minutes, preferably an hour or longer, so that oil can form.

2. You may have come to your own conclusion as to skin type based upon misinformation or by identifying yourself with a product.

Here's a common mistake: Ms. Skin Care Consumer is looking through a magazine and sees an ad for a moisturizer. She reads it and decides that yes, indeed, she needs a moisturizer. She then takes the next step and assumes that she has dry skin. This kind of skin typing by product identification is done by just about everybody at one time or another.

Perhaps the more typical version of this is the woman who has normal skin, but as a teenager had mild acne. She responded by using products to dry out her skin. Now ten or fifteen years later, she assumes, therefore, that she still has oily skin and is still using the same products.

3. You may have used too many of the wrong products and created your own case of mismanaged skin, and it now mimics another skin type.

Many young women with normal skin have jumped on the dry skin bandwagon and used moisturizers and cleansers that were designed for mature skin. This scenario can then play itself out in two different ways. Sometimes when the pores get clogged, the women end up visiting their cosmetics counter, where they are told that they have oily skin, and they begin an oily skin regimen. Or, the pores don't get that clogged, but the skin starts looking caked and dull, and the skin care consumer sees this as an indication that her skin is getting dryer.

4. You may have had your skin typed by computer or machine, but the technician may not have known how to evaluate the results.

The computers used by the skin care companies are quite efficient when it comes to typing skin, but it is a person who most often interprets the results.

A Test to Help You Determine Your Skin Type

The biggest mistake that most of us make in determining our skin type is in just not taking enough time or care to do it properly. The first thing to do is to think about it. Asking yourself the following questions and thinking about the answers will help you determine your skin type.

1. What skin type are your natural parents and other relatives?
This is an important question to consider because skin type, like so many other things, is genetically influenced.

2. In what country were your ancestors born?
If your grandparents or great-grandparents came from Italy, Greece, or the Middle East, you have a better chance of having oily skin than if they came from the British Isles, Scandinavia, or northern Europe.

3. What is your skin tone?
If you are very fair, with blonde hair and blue eyes, it's unlikely that you have oily skin. If you have dark hair and olive-toned skin, your skin is probably not going to be dry.

4. How often do you have to wash your hair?
Women with dry skin most often have dry hair that can go several days without washing. Women with oily skin have oily hair that may need a daily shampoo. And women with combination-type skin often have moderately oily hair.

5. How large are your pores?
Women with dry skin usually have very small, barely visible pores. Women with normal skin have small pores. Women with oily skin have large pores. And women with combination-type skin have large pores in their T-zones and normal-sized pores elsewhere.

6. When you wear foundation, blusher, or any other form of makeup, how often does it need to be reapplied?
Women with oily skin complain, rightly so, that the oil on their faces causes makeup to "disappear" too quickly. If you have dry skin, foundation and blusher will have a long face life.

A Common Mistake in Determining Skin Type: The Perpetually Adolescent Skin-Type Myth Just about every teenager has oily skin. The statistics on teenage acne say that at least 80 percent, possibly more, of all adolescents have some experience with acne. Does this mean that all of these teenagers turn into adults with oily skin? Absolutely not. Most of them turn into adults with normal or combination-type skin. But many women aren't aware of this. I have known several women with normal skin who were absolutely convinced that they had oily skin. Why? Because they had had mild acne and mildly oily skin as teenagers.

Here is what typically happens with skin type as a woman goes from adolescence to young adulthood:

· If, as a teenager, your skin was very oily and you experienced moderate to severe acne flare-ups that occurred on the cheeks as well as in the T-zone, then, as an adult, you probably still have *oily* skin.
· If, as a teenager, your skin was moderately oily and you experienced moderate acne flare-ups and pimples that were mostly confined to the area of the T-zone, then, as an adult, you probably have *combination*-type skin.
· If, as a teenager, your skin was mildly oily, and you experienced mild acne-type flare-ups and occasional pimples, then, as an adult, you probably have *normal* skin.
· If, as a teenager, you rarely had a pimple and never went out to purchase a tube of over-the-counter acne preparations, then, as an adult, you probably have *dry* skin.

Why Most Women over Forty Have Dry Skin: Using Age and Some Statistics About Sebum Production to Help You Determine Your Skin Type We all like to think that we are a little bit different from everyone else, and we are. But there are also amazing similarities, and one of these is the way in which we age.

Whether our skin is oily or dry is determined by how much oil is produced by our sebaceous glands. How much oil our sebaceous glands produce is very much determined by hormones, and hormones, in turn, rise and wane depending upon our individual ages.

What does this mean? Female adolescents have the highest rate of sebum production. It goes down substantially by the time we reach twenty, and pretty much stays at the same level for the next twenty years. By the time we hit forty, however, sebum production has decreased. And, after menopause, which for many women is in the late forties or early fifties, sebum production takes a real nosedive.

This reduced sebum production spells dry skin for most women as they near menopause. And as we get older, our skin gets even drier and requires better and more efficient moisturizing.

If You Are Between the Ages of Twenty and Forty, You Probably Have Normal or Combination-Type Skin: Avoiding the Myth of Prematurely Dry Skin It seems as though the ads in just about every magazine published for women are telling us that we should worry about the kind of little fine lines that form on dry skin. You pick up a magazine and notice an ad for a skin care product. The copy is talking about little fine lines that are beginning to form. The model, who is worried about these lines, looks as though she is twenty, and she has no lines whatsoever. You are closer to thirty and have a few lines you are not too crazy about under your eyes. What are you to think? If she has dry skin, what on earth do you have? Cardboard, that's what!

Does that scenario sound familiar? Skin care ads push so many products for dry skin that it's understandable that the average woman is convinced that she must also have dry skin.

If you are between the ages of twenty and thirty-five, the chances are that your sebaceous glands are producing enough oil so that you have normal or combination-type skin. This does not mean that you don't need a moisturizer, but it does mean that you do not have dry skin, and you don't need overkill skin care regimens designed for dry and mature skin.

Take a Good Look at Your Skin

You should be able to differentiate between dry, oily, and normal skin without too much trouble, but you do need some form of magnification. I prefer using a magnifying glass and a mirror. Some women use just a magnifying mirror. Three hours before you examine your skin you should wash off all old moisturizers and creams as well as makeup, using a mild, nondrying soap. Do not apply any new moisturizers, makeup, or creams. Here's what you should see:

· *Normal skin.* Normal skin should appear moist and smooth, but not oily or shiny. Pores are visible without magnification, but they are not large, and they are rarely, if ever, clogged. The texture of normal skin is not porcelain-fine, but it is also not coarse or thick. Normal skin will typically not have any acne scars or any comedones or blemishes.
· *Dry skin.* Dry skin often appears very thin and translucent. The pores are hardly visible and are definitely not clogged. Very dry skin can appear flaky and cracked or chapped, particularly around the sides of

the cheeks. There will often be small fine lines around the mouth and eyes. Any blemishes that exist are likely to be caused by sensitivity.

· *Oily skin.* Oily skin often feels oily when you touch it. The pores, which are large and visible, may be clogged. There may be a few small acne scars from adolescence. The skin, particularly on the forehead and chin, may appear shiny.

· *Oily problem skin.* Oily problem skin usually feels very oily. The pores are large and visible, and only the most conscientious care can keep them from appearing clogged. The texture is often coarse or thick, and there will probably be several acne scars, a reminder of the most severe acne flare-ups. The chances are good that even as an adult there will be some comedones and blemishes that require treatment.

· *Combination-type skin.* Combination-type skin is exactly what it sounds like—a mixed bag. When you look at it, you will probably see visible pores that are not clogged on the forehead and cheeks and pores that are clogged on the sides of the nose and chin. The skin on the cheeks may appear normally moist or even dry. The skin on the nose and on the bridge of the nose will probably appear oily.

A Simple Test for Skin Type

If you are still unsure of your skin type, here's the best test I know. All you need is a mild soap, some blotting paper and a little bit of time. You can use either facial blotting paper, cigarette paper, or onion skin typing paper. Whichever kind you use, it should be cut into four one-inch-square parts:

1. Wash your face with lukewarm water and a mild soap, such as Dove or Lowila. Rinse your skin by splashing it at least fifteen times, again with lukewarm or tepid water. When you are finished, don't apply any moisturizer, even if your face feels dry, and wait at least three hours.
2. Mark your four pieces of paper as follows: forehead, cheek, nose, chin.
3. One at a time, hold the appropriate papers on your forehead, cheek, nose, and chin for a count of ten. Make sure it's a slow count.
4. Take the papers into a good light and look at them.

Any papers that are dry or unmarked by oil indicate where your skin is dry.

If any of the papers come away with a very faint, barely discernible oil residue, it indicates where your skin is normal.

If any papers come away with a slight, but definitely discernible, oil residue, it indicates where your skin is oily.

If any papers come away with a heavy oil residue, it indicates where your skin is very oily.

With true dry skin, all of the papers will be dry. If you have typical T-zone combination-type skin, one or more of the papers marked forehead, nose, and chin will be oily. The paper marked cheek will be dry.

Black Skin—Special Considerations

Black women have the best chances of maintaining healthy, unwrinkled skin for most of their lives. This is because black skin has more natural melanin, which gives it much greater protection from ultraviolet light. Black skin is therefore less likely to experience the ravages of photoaging. The average white woman will have wrinkling and fine lines on her face by the time she reaches forty; the average black woman may have an unlined face until she is fifty or sixty. Much of this kind of wrinkling is caused by sun damage.

The black skin care consumer has to realize, however, that the level of protection that she receives is dependent upon the amount of melanin in her skin. If you are a light-skinned black, your skin needs as much sunscreen protection as a white woman with olive skin tone.

Black women always have to be aware of the possibility of problems caused by pigmentation. Black skin is prone to exaggerated pigment responses, and increased or decreased pigmentation can occur following even minor cutaneous reactions.

One special problem that black women have to be aware of is a condition called melasma. This is hyperpigmentation that can occur primarily on the sun-exposed area of the face. Because it happens mostly with women, some experts feel it may be associated with hormonal conditions and can be connected to oral contraceptives or pregnancy. Melasma seems to have a genetic predisposition. If the melanization is brought on by sun exposure, prevention is the best solution, and a sunscreen with a high SPF is recommended. Melasma, incidentally, happens with both white and black skin.

Other than the melanin content and the pigmentary differences, there doesn't seem to be much difference between black skin and white. The black skin care consumer has about the same chances of having oily, dry, or combination-type skin. However, if you have very dark skin, oily skin may appear to be oilier than it really is because of the way light is reflected off of the darker tones. And dry skin may appear to be drier because the flaky dead skin cells can give a grayish dull hue in contrast to the darker tone.

Black women with acne-prone skin should take into account that black skin probably has a greater tendency for scarring, and a low-level acne flare-up has to be treated with special care. The same type of extra sensitivity is true when it comes to irritants or allergens. Black skin is always prone to exaggerated pigment responses, and the slightest irritation can have an effect on the pigment. For this reason, black women have to be particularly careful of any type of harsh products that can damage the skin. Harsh abrasives, for example, can be a problem, particularly if they are used with a great deal of zeal.

Black women with oily skin should take extra precautions not to use products that might clog the pores and precipitate acne flare-ups. As a rule, it's a good idea to stick with noncomedegenic moisturizers. Acne has to be treated with great care and whenever possible should really be monitored by a knowledgeable dermatologist.

The dermatologists to whom I spoke who were well informed about black skin stressed gentle care at all times. Also, although much of the literature on sun care tends to indicate that darker-skinned black women do not need sunscreens, they felt that even dark-skinned black women should use sunscreens for two reasons: (1) To avoid pigment changes such as vitiligo, melasma, etc. (2) Although the darker tones of black skin are pretty well protected from UVB sun damage, there is no guarantee of protection against UVA, which reaches further into the skin. UVA may have long term effects that are damaging, and not enough is known about UVA and skin cancer. The feeling is that all of us are living longer, more active lives. Even if you don't run the risk of an immediate sunburn, why run the risk of a more serious problem later on.

Sensitive Skin

Recently I met a woman who claims that she breaks out from every form of moisturizer or cream she has ever tried. Her skin is very dry, but she can't use anything without getting some form of dermatitis. She also said that she is allergic to wool and to most soaps, as well as just about every perfume she has ever tried.

She is obviously an exception. However, some women seem to have skin that is easily irritated; itching, burning, chafing, stinging, and other words that indicate skin discomfort are all too familiar. Technically, any skin type can be sensitive, and although there is a tendency to believe that the fair-skinned and porcelain-thin-skinned woman will be most reactive to a whole range of irritants, this is not necessarily true.

Some of the most common irritants such as cold air, dry air, and ultraviolet light are environmental. Many women are truly disturbed by skin that becomes chafed or chapped or dried-out looking every time they are exposed to an unruly wind or an overactive central heating system. Nonenvironmental materials that can bring on contact dermatitis are known as allergens or skin sensitizers.

Allergic contact dermatitis is the direct result of being exposed to an allergen. Primary irritants are those substances to which your skin reacts on first exposure. This can happen, for example, if a very strong alkali or acid comes in contact with your skin and produces a burn or some other serious response.

Secondary irritants, which is what we are ordinarily concerned about when we discuss skin care products, are milder and will normally provoke a response only when your skin has had time to build up an allergic type reaction. It may be difficult to understand how a product that may have been used for months suddenly causes a problem. But that's what an allergy is. It doesn't happen the first time you come in contact with the allergen—your body has to become sensitized.

An acute allergic reaction is one that happens within minutes after exposure. These reactions can be very extreme and, sometimes, even life-threatening. This can happen if the allergen is injected, as in a drug; inhaled, as in fumes or plant pollen; or eaten, as in shellfish or strawberries; or absorbed through the skin if the substance is one that can be absorbed.

Reactions to skin care products are rarely acute. More often it is what is known as a delayed reaction and takes at least an hour or so to develop. A cosmetic product can produce many different kinds of reactions, such as stinging, burning, itching, drying, and scaling, as well as eruptions such as rashes or hives.

Recently, dermatologists have become more sensitive to the fact that some women react badly to just about everything that touches the skin. Dr. Albert Kligman, of the University of Pennsylvania, whom many consider to be the most distinguished dermatologist in the country, recently spoke to the Society of Cosmetic Chemists and said that he now realizes that there are women who can't put anything on their faces without a reaction, something which he once treated with skepticism as he did the complaints of patients about invisible itches and irritations. He stated that early inflammatory events cannot always be perceived by the naked eye and said, "As I've gotten older, however, I've come to realize the importance of what the patient is saying, even though nothing is visible to the naked eye. We should trust our patients more and our eyes less."

Skin that is easily irritated is often referred to as *problem-sensitive skin.* Unfortunately, this type of reaction is sometimes exacerbated or induced by cosmetic products, and a recent study seemed to indicate that some of the heaviest users of cosmetic products were among those with the most sensitive skin.

Problem-sensitive skin is often addressed by the cosmetics industry by introducing a whole range of products directed at the woman who is trying to find some level of "hypoallergenic" in the products she buys. However, when someone has become *sensitive* to a whole range of ingredients, it becomes increasingly difficult to find products that are not potentially troublesome.

It is not unusual for women to find that simultaneous exposure to several potentially irritating factors is what causes skin sensitivity or dermatitis. For example, if my friend Marianne bathes in very hot water on a cold day, applies perfume, and then puts on a wool sweater, she gets contact dermatitis wherever the wool has touched her skin. Take away the perfume or the hot bath or the very cold weather, and the wool doesn't bother her at all.

Frequently, weather and environmental factors play a vital role in skin sensitivity. Winter, which brings the combination of cold air and central heating, seems to have a particularly bad effect on sensitive skin problems.

A Rash by Any Other Name

Over the years, I've spoken to many women who had skin eruptions that seemed to have some sort of an allergic basis, but they were unable to pinpoint the cause. If this happens to you, you should get yourself to a competent dermatologist, and together you should try to sort out the problem. Some of the questions the doctor might ask you include:

- Your occupation. You might be having an occupationally related skin problem, particularly if you work in or around certain chemicals.
- Your immediate personal environment.
- Do you have plants, pets, woolen rugs, or a roommate who develops photographs in your bathroom?
- Are you taking any drugs, prescription or nonprescription? Drugs, even commonplace ones such as aspirin, have been implicated in skin eruptions.
- Any previous treatment, either from another doctor, or self-prescribed. This includes all salves, lotions, etc.
- Cosmetics used. Don't leave out face creams, body lotions, etc., even if you have been using them for years.
- Illnesses or physical conditions, such as pregnancy or menopause. Another illness might be implicated, or your hormones may be involved.
- Foods. Everyone always assumes a rash is food-related, but food is not always the cause. When it is, some common foods that have been implicated include seafoods, nuts, fruits, berries, onions, and garlic.

Emotions and Your Skin

Your emotions are another factor that one should consider if your skin starts reacting strangely. Yes, it's true, it's true. When some people are upset, they get hives. Certainly, when it comes to emotions and illness, it is very difficult to generalize. However, there does seem to be new evidence that indicates that outbreaks of some dermatological conditions can be brought on or exacerbated by emotional factors. I haven't seen any real figures on this, but it is probably quite unusual for one's emotional state to trigger a dermatological condition unless the tendency for the problem already exists. For example, it is unlikely that being upset will give you acne, but if you already have it, emotional stress can make your skin act up. The same is true of seborrheic dermatitis, atopic dermatitis, all forms of eczema except contact, and hand dermatitis.

Most experts agree, however, that if you and your dermatologist decide that you have a stress-related dermatological outbreak, it is still important to continue to treat it medically. And you should never decide, on your own, that a recurring dermatological problem is solely emotionally based.

Even a condition that appears as disarmingly simple as hives can have a more complex diagnosis.

The Skin Around Your Eyes

The skin of the eye area, which is highly elastic, is thinner than that found on the rest of the body. If you gently touch the upper or lower eyelid, you can feel how thin and moveable the skin feels compared to that on rest of the face. Because the skin around the eyes is so sensitive, this is often the first place to reveal telltale signs of aging. Consequently, a wide variety of cosmetic skin care products are marketed to appeal to the many women concerned about the appearance of the skin around the eyes. But many women are confused and often fail to distinguish between those conditions that are physiological or medical in origin and those that are cosmetic.

The most common problems affecting the eye area are:

Puffiness is most often caused by edema, which is the retaining of excess fluid by the body. If you are bothered by puffy eyes, excess fluid is being held in the subcutaneous spaces around the eye. Because more fluid accumulates when one is lying down, you may notice that your eyes are most likely to look puffy when you first wake up. As the day progresses, the head is held higher than the body and drainage naturally occurs.

Puffiness is sometimes attributed to allergens such as smoke, animal dander, and pollen, and many women say that they are most aware of swollen eyes when they are menstruating.

Sometimes a sinus infection (chronic or acute) or a postnasal drip will aggravate a tendency toward swollen-looking eyes. In these cases, the solution can be found by treating the medical condition.

Puffiness can also be caused by rubbing or irritating the eyes, and, as many women know, crying is an almost certain way to produce puffy swollen eyes.

Bags are caused by slack skin and *fatty deposits* that, unlike puffiness, do not disappear. The eyes normally have fat pockets—two in the upper eyelid and three in the lower. Medical experts believe that a tendency towards fatty deposits is inherited. Some women begin to show signs of these deposits while they are very young, but fatty deposits typically don't occur until after forty, when a weakness in the supporting muscle structure allows the fat to push itself out. Although fatty deposits can occur in either the upper or the bottom lid, they seem to be more common on the bottom.

Dark circles can have several different causes. In some women, fat deposits cast a yellowish hue. In others, the network of tiny blood vessels is very close to the thin skin surface and provides a bluish tone to the area. This is particularly noticeable when the skin is exceptionally pale and thin in the eye area, putting even more emphasis on the dark circles. Skin color, of course, is always related to melanin, and some people have more melanin under their eyes than others do. However, it is important to know that there is a correlation between stress and the production of melanin, and dark circles can become more pronounced when one is fatigued or under stress. Because dark circles can also be an indicator of medical problems such as anemia, it's a good idea to rule out the possibility of an underlying physical problem before looking for cosmetic solutions.

Crowsfeet, as we all know, are the tiny lines that form at the corners of the eyes. They are made more pronounced every time we smile or frown or squint. Women with very prominent crowsfeet probably spent too many unprotected hours in the sun.

Gels, Creams, Balms and Other Cosmetic Products Designed for the Area Around the Eyes Eye cream is the traditional product, but within the last few years, the cosmetics industry has begun introducing new types of products for the eye area.

Products that are designed to reduce puffiness will often include botanicals such as comfrey, marigold, and chamomile because in herbology these ingredients are associated with dehydrating properties.

Products that are marketed to temporarily firm skin and improve the appearance of bags and sags sometimes include botanical extracts with astringent properties such as low concentrations of witch hazel. Some other botanicals believed to have an astringent effect include horsetail, blackberry, and elderflower. These products may also include protein extracts.

Products designed to moisturize and soften the skin, improving the appearance of wrinkles or crowsfeet, will typically include ingredients such as collagen, petrolatum, hyaluronic acid, and glycerin.

When shopping for eye products you should be very clear about what your particular problem is and what you want to do about it. Otherwise you may purchase the wrong type of product.

Defining your particular eye problem before you visit the store and determining what sort of product you want can save you time and money. Many companies manufacture different types of eye products at different prices, designed for different skin types or different problems. For example, Estée Lauder markets

Estée Lauder Swiss Eye Cream. Some of the ingredients are hydroxylated lanolin, soluble collagen extract, butyl stearate, and mineral oil.

Estée Lauder Maximum Eye Care. Some of the ingredients are soluble collagen extract, sodium RNA, and emulsifying wax.

Estée Lauder Eyezone Repair Gel. Some of the ingredients are tissue matrix extract, cholesteric esters, glycerine, and retinyl palmitate.

Other companies manufacture a wide variety of moisturizing eye products, and companies such as Clarins, whose promotional literature stresses plant extracts, specialize in products that are high in botanicals.

If you have a tendency to allergic reactions from cosmetics ingredients, the eyes are particularly vulnerable. Typical reactions are itching, burning, or tearing. Preservatives and fragrances are the most frequently cited allergens.

Avoiding Ultraviolet Light Is the Best Protection Against Crowsfeet! Much of the wrinkling and loss of skin elasticity around the eyes is directly attributed to sun damage. Protecting the delicate skin around the eyes from solar damage is the best way to prevent crowsfeet and loose skin around your eyes.

And don't forget that sunlight and ultraviolet radiation is bad not only for the skin, but also for the eyes. For maximum eye protection, always wear sunglasses that absorb almost all radiation in the UVA and UVB range. When buying prescription sunglasses, ask your optician or optometrist to prescribe the appropriate lenses. With nonprescription eyeglasses, be certain that the lens meets the standards set by the American National Standards Institute. Glasses that meet these standards should have an appropriate notation.

Medical Solutions for Cosmetic Problems Most members of the medical profession feel that cosmetic products offer only temporary solutions to skin problems and emphasize medical treatments such as cosmetic surgery for bags and sags and collagen injections for wrinkles. Perhaps the treatment getting the most attention these days is the use of Retin-A to attempt to reverse crowsfeet caused by sun damage.

6

Understanding Your Skin Type

Dry Skin—What Is It?

The stratum corneum, or uppermost layer of the epidermis, is normally made up of 10 to 20 percent water. If the water level goes below 10 percent, the cells become parched and can actually appear brittle and scaly. When that happens, you have dry skin.

Dry skin is confusing, because it can come and go, depending upon environmental factors. Also, there are many degrees of dry skin. If you have very dry skin, it sometimes becomes a medical condition because very dry skin is acutely uncomfortable and may itch or become inflamed. Garden-variety dry skin, which becomes more pronounced as we age, usually starts to become apparent sometime after the twentieth birthday, as the amount of natural oil secretion begins to decrease. If you have a tendency toward dry skin, it may first become noticeable on your arms and lower legs because there are fewer oil glands in these areas.

If dry skin is your primary problem, water, or moisture, is the ingredient that is missing. This lack of moisture is, however, traditionally associated with sebaceous glands that are not producing enough sebum to keep the top layer of skin soft and moisturized. Here's why: Sebum by itself does not produce moist, well-hydrated skin. However, if the skin cells are all hydrated and plumped up, sebum, which forms a protective oily film over the skin, will serve as a barrier to keep the moisture in place.

Dry skin, then, is missing two ingredients: moisture to keep the cells plump and hydrated, and an oily film to keep the moisture from evaporating.

What's good about dry skin? Small pores, that's what. If you have dry skin all over your face, including your T-zone, it is unlikely that you will have to worry about large pores that so easily get clogged.

The other good thing about dry skin? As annoying as it can be, more often than not it is a purely cosmetic problem and can be remedied with enough moisture.

Different Kinds of Dry Skin

Caused by Environmental Factors Everyone gets dry skin once in a while. It is often associated with environmental conditions. Too much time in the sun will dry the skin. So will an overheated room with low humidity. A cold wind, a dry day, a frosty snow—all of these environmental conditions will cause the skin to dry.

Relative humidity is an important factor in how dry or moist our skin is. If you live in a city with a high relative humidity, your skin will tend to retain its moisture; if you are in an environment that is drying, such as an airplane, your skin cells will start to look and feel dryer.

Women who live in states that are exceptionally dry often complain of skin that feels as though it is pulled taut. Several women from western states told me that during summers when there have been droughts, particularly when there are forest fires within a hundred miles, their skin starts to feel totally parched. And, of course, women who live in cities where there is a great deal of rain rarely have that complaint.

Caused by Inappropriate Care Dry skin is sometimes something we do to ourselves. Here are some of the ways in which we create or aggravate dry skin.

· Using facial treatments that are drying, such as drying masks, scrubs, or alcohol-based astringents.

· Exposing the skin to irritating fabrics such as heavy woolens or clothing that has been washed in harsh detergents.
· Washing with water that is too hot or with soap that is too harsh.
· Drinking too little water and neglecting to replace fluid loss in your body.

There is another type of "false" dry skin that is cosmetically induced. In these instances, the cosmetics consumer caused sebaceous glands to behave in a somewhat "sluggish" fashion and interfered with normal functioning by applying heavy creams and lotions that clog up the pores and create a false type of dry skin.

Associated with Maturing and Aging As we age, our skin becomes dryer. The term mature skin has become almost synonymous with dry skin. Remember, as we get older, hormonal changes slow down the sebum output so that there are fewer natural oils to help bind moisture to the skin. Also, the skin naturally becomes thinner and is thus less able to retain moisture. And there is a decrease in natural mucopolysaccharides that help bind moisture to the skin.

Associated with Premature Aging and Sun Damage If you expose your unprotected skin to the ultraviolet rays of the sun, you will experience sun damage and dry skin. There is no way around it.

Oily Skin—What Is It?

Oily skin is usually something you come by genetically. If members of your family are from the Mediterranean area or the Middle East, your chances of having oily skin are dramatically increased. Although it is not always the case, the typical woman with oily skin has dark hair and an olive complexion. It's a mistake to assume that oily skin automatically means acne; it doesn't. Oily skin can be totally blemish-free.

Oily skin is the result of very active sebaceous glands. Sebaceous glands, in turn, are affected by hormones. This means that every time your body goes through a hormonal change, your skin is affected. Adolescence is the time for really oily skin. Other times: Typically women have a surge of hormonal activity about a week to ten days before they menstruate, and this can create oily skin problems. If you get pregnant, you may actually have less oily skin during the last six months of your pregnancy. Then, a few months after you give birth, when the hormones have gone back to normal, the sebaceous glands may become temporarily even more active.

Sebaceous gland activity can change according to the seasons. Some women feel that their skin is less oily in the summer; other women respond badly to the sun and have acne flare-ups when they are exposed to it.

The good news about oily skin is that as one gets older, and hormonal activity slows down, the average woman with oily skin develops fewer acne-type breakouts. Her skin becomes closer to normal. Because sebum keeps the skin soft and supple and protects it against moisture loss, women with oily skin typically have fewer fine lines. They are often spared all those tiny wrinkles that one associates with dry skin.

Comedones and Acne-Type Breakouts—The Worst Thing About Oily Skin

Comedone is a fairly fancy word that dermatologists use to describe acne-type breakouts. Unless it becomes a serious affliction, most of us are more likely to think of them as zits or pimples.

Comedones tend to occur primarily on the face, back, chest, and shoulders. I think it's important to point out that if you have one or two pimples, you may have oily skin, but you do not necessarily have acne. However, I think it is also important to point out that if you repeatedly develop comedones, you probably have a mild case of acne and should be treating it accordingly.

A dermatologist makes a diagnosis of acne when there is a finding of several acne lesions, usually of a different type located on the face and body. Here are the different types of acne lesions:

· *Comedone (Whitehead or Blackhead).* A comedone, the most common manifestation of acne, is the primary acne lesion. This lesion, which is not inflamed, is the direct result of sebum, dead skin cells, and bacteria clogging up the hair follicle, or pore, as we sometimes call it.

There are two separate forms of comedones:

Blackheads are also known as open comedones. They are easily recognizable for most of us because when you look at a blackhead you see a pore that is clogged with a dark substance. This dark color, as I'm sure you know by now, does not come from dirt, but from melanin in the skin.

Whiteheads are also called closed comedones. They are sometimes harder to see and can appear as simply pale, shiny, slightly elevated bumps. They are called closed comedones because the opening is not visible to the naked eye. Typically, the closed comedones either rupture or become inflamed lesions, which are known to dermatologists as papules, pustules, or nodules and to the layman as pimples. The second form a whitehead can take is to develop into an open comedone or blackhead. This occurs when dead skin cells that accumulate cause the whitehead to open and become a blackhead.

If your acne-type breakout consists of only blackheads and whiteheads, it is considered noninflammatory acne.

· *Papule.* This is a small inflamed lesion that forms from a ruptured closed comedone. It is probably the smallest lesion (or pimple) that is formed; it can either develop into a larger lesion, known as a pustule, or it will spontaneously clear up. If it clears up, the process typically takes two to three weeks.

· *Pustule.* The next stage in the process of an inflamed acne lesion is a pustule. It is more inflamed than a papule and is filled with pus. Many pustules are superficial and will start clearing up within a few days with no scarring effects. A more severe postule, however, can take two to six weeks to go away, and scarring often results.

· *Nodule.* A nodule is a larger, and more inflamed, pus-filled acne lesion. Nodules, which are deep-seated lesions, are often quite painful, and scarring is a common result. The term "cystic acne" is sometimes used to refer to the condition that exists when these nodules become inflamed.

· *Cyst.* This is defined as the largest and most uncomfortable of the acne lesions.

Who Gets Acne

Acne, which is associated with oily skin, is a condition that usually first makes its presence felt during adolescence. As a matter of fact, the disease is sometimes one of the first manifestations of puberty, and, according to some statistics, affects nearly 80 percent of the teenage population at one time or another. Fortunately for most of us, the majority of these cases are mild and self-limited. However, for some women, adolescence is only the beginning of a battle against acne problem skin. If you have acne-prone skin, it probably doesn't comfort you to be told that in all likelihood the condition appears much worse to you than to those around you. Everyone with acne seems to be acutely aware of every new blemish and comedone. Perhaps this is because the disease most often makes its presence felt during those teenage years when sense of self is more apt to be bound up in appearance and image.

It might be interesting to examine some results of a study that presented estimates of the prevalence of facial acne in teenagers aged twelve to seventeen nationwide by age, sex, and geographic region. It was published in 1976 by the U.S. Department of Health, Education, and Welfare.

- Of the teenagers studied, 28.3 percent had moderate to severe facial acne.
- Although facial acne is as prevalent in girls as in boys, the condition tends to start earlier in young males and to be more severe.
- Both black and white teenagers have acne at about the same rate, but acne tends to be more severe in white skin.
- Facial acne was found to be slightly more prevalent among adolescents who were living in the South and West as compared to those living in the Northeast or Midwest, but there seemed to be no consistent pattern in differences between urban and rural youths.
- Those who rate themselves as being in good health had slightly less acne than those who consider themselves in fair or poor health.
- Those who believe that they are nervous in temperament had more acne than those who did not.
- In these young people there appeared to be some correlation between their acne conditions and the education levels of their parents; their acne rates go down as their parental education levels go up.
- There did not appear to be any correlation between family income level and acne prevalence.
- Acne levels were higher in those young males whose parents said they tended to eat too much as opposed to those who said their offspring ate too little.
- There was a consistent pattern of acne increasing with the degree of development of secondary sex characteristics in both boys and girls.

How a Comedone Develops

Although the underlying cause of acne has yet to be discovered, a great deal is known about the way in which it behaves and develops.

Take a look at the following diagram of the philosebaceous unit and note the sebaceous gland and sebaceous follicle that are connected to the surface of the skin by the follicular canal. The openings of these sebaceous follicles are the openings we call pores.

The sebaceous gland, as you know, produces sebum, which we lay people usually refer to as oil. If you have oily skin, and most people with acne have *very* oily skin, it is because you have very active sebaceous glands, and they are emptying their secretions into the sebaceous follicles.

The main difference between sebaceous follicles and hair follicles, by the way, is the absence of a fully developed hair. If you have oily hair, your sebaceous glands are every bit as active on your scalp, but the oil is emptying out into a hair follicle, and the hair acts as a conveyor, or helper, for the oil that pours out onto the scalp. The sebaceous follicle, which usually has only an undeveloped hair, has no such helper, and the oil is on its own in terms of finding its way onto the skin.

The next important thing to remember about these sebaceous follicles is that the top layer of the skin, the stratum corneum, forms a lining for the sebaceous follicle exactly as it does for the exterior of the skin that we see. In other words, the stratum corneum continues down into the pore and back up again. This lining is not as thick as it is on the exterior of the skin, but it is there nonetheless, and it behaves exactly in the same way as it does on the surface. New skin cells form, and old dead ones come to the top in order to be shed.

The other thing you need to know about these sebaceous follicles is that they are ideal resting places for certain forms of bacteria. The bacteria were originally named corynebacterium acnes because it was believed that they were responsible for acne. We now know that everyone has these bacteria whether or not they have acne. These bacteria are anaerobic bacteria, which means that they live only in the absence of oxygen.

Sebum and Acne

No discussion of acne would be complete without at least mentioning sebum, the oily substance that seems to be the exacerbating factor in the

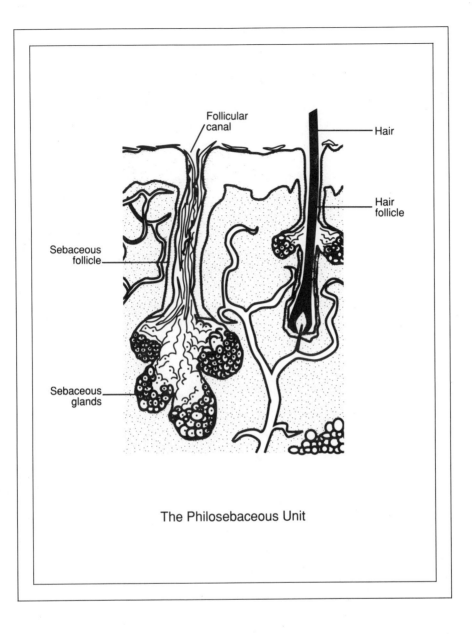

The Philosebaceous Unit

problem. Sebum is made up of glycerides and free fatty acids, wax esters, squalene, cholesteryl esters, and cholesterol, and it prevents moisture loss from the skin.

For a long time, people thought that sebum production was dependent upon outside factors such as temperature or how often the face was washed, but researchers are now fairly certain that sebum production is continuous and uniform. It has nothing to do with how frequently or infrequently you wash your face, and although heat may cause the sebum to reach the skin's surface more rapidly, it is not believed that it speeds up the actual production.

How much or how little sebum is produced is dependent upon age and sex as well as skin type. Typically, sebum production is highest in adolescence in both men and women. In adulthood, it is higher in men than it is in women. Then, in women, sebum production drops sharply after menopause (ages fifty to fifty-nine). In men, sebum production stays fairly constant until the sixties.

Why Do Some People Have Acne and Others Do Not?

It seems like a logical question. We all have sebaceous glands and the sebum that they produce, as well as the anaerobic bacteria that live in our sebaceous follicles. We all also have skin cells that go through the process of cell renewal and are shed into the sebaceous follicles. Why, then, do some people get acne while others do not?

When someone does not have acne, the skin cells within the sebaceous gland are shed and are brought to the surface of the skin through the pore along with the sebum that is being produced by the sebaceous gland. When someone does have acne, the system, simply put, doesn't work, but no one is quite sure precisely why.

In individuals with acne, there is a speeding up of cell turnover within the sebaceous follicles, and there is an alteration in the pattern of keratinization. This means that more and more dead skin cells are being shed into the sebaceous follicle.

Individuals with acne also produce more sebum than those without acne; people with severe acne produce more than those with mild acne.

When someone has acne, the skin cells clump up in the follicle, where they are joined with the sebum and the bacteria that normally grow in the sebaceous follicle. Together, they comprise the material that clogs the pores and causes comedones to form.

All Acne Is Not Alike

There are several different kinds of acne, including:

- True acne, which is also known as *acne vulgaris.* Although this, the most common form of acne, is usually considered a disease of adolescence, it may linger until the thirties or even forties. In fact, some cases begin long after adolescence. True acne usually begins with open or closed comedones on the forehead or chin before spreading to the cheeks.
- *Acne conglobata* is a more severe and chronic form of acne vulgaris, often with large and painful lesions occurring on the face, back, and chest as well as on the upper arms, neck, thighs, and buttocks. Males are more apt to be affected than females. Acne conglobata most often occurs between eighteen and thirty and can continue, off and on, for a good number of years.
- There is an even more acute form of acne known as *acne fulminans,* which is a rare and more severe form of the disease, in which the main lesions are inflamed nodules. Acne fulminans can be accompanied by fever, anemia, and swollen joints.

There is no special word that tells someone how much or how little acne she has. The same word, acne, applies for all degrees of severity, but in reality acne can be very mild, or very serious, and the two extremes of the disease can be quite different in terms of both appearance and treatment.

Acne is usually graded.

- Grade 1 acne is the mildest form of the disease. In mild acne there may be only a scattering of noninflamed open and closed comedones.
- Grade 2 acne is the typical case of teenage acne. It consists of open and closed comedones as well as papules and pustules. Although it can be very discomforting to the person who has it, it does not normally produce serious scarring.
- Grade 3 acne is moderately severe and there are numerous small pustules as well as an occasional larger lesion, and it will normally affect the chest, neck, shoulders, and back as well as the face.
- Grade 4 acne is the most serious form of acne, referred to as acne conglobata.

Hormones and Acne

It would appear that hormones play a crucial role in precipitating acne. This seems plausible since acne is so often associated with the hormonal changes of puberty. There have also been some studies that have shown that plasma testosterone levels are higher in those who have acne during early puberty. It is also known that acne can be brought on or exacerbated when someone receives hormone treatments. As a matter of fact, in many cases of adult-onset acne the cautious physician will insist upon looking into the possibility of some type of underlying hormonal problem.

What happens at puberty is that the process by which the hormone androgen is secreted is speeded up. Although androgen is known as the male sex hormone, both men and women secrete it. In men, androgen comes mainly from the testes. In women, it comes from the ovaries and adrenal glands. Testosterone, the most potent androgen, circulates through the body and is converted into dehydroepiandrosterone, which is the insanely long name of the form of testosterone that stimulates the sebaceous glands to get larger and produce more oil.

One would assume from all of this that acne patients would have elevated levels of testosterone, but in males this is not the case, and the slight elevation found in some studies on women does not seem to be enough to create the acne problem.

What some researchers now believe is that it is not the level of androgens that is creating the problem, but the degree of sensitivity. In other words, acne patients may have sebaceous glands that are extrasensitive to testosterone.

Women's Hormonal Fluctuation By definition, women go through several hormonal changes that may affect or precipitate acne. They include:

· *Monthly menstrual cycle.* If you are an acne-prone woman, the chances are very good that you have acne flare-ups that somehow correspond to your menstrual cycle. Typically, these acne-type eruptions occur about a week before menstruation begins. This correlation is missed by many women since it sort of happens some place in the middle of their cycle, but it has been estimated that 60 to 70 percent of women with acne have some form of premenstrual flare-up.
· *Pregnancy.* The hormones of pregnancy may actually alleviate acne, and a pregnant woman's acne often clears up after the first three

months of pregnancy. When you're pregnant, your body is being flooded with extra estrogen and the estrogen–androgen ratio changes. This seems to have the effect of making acne-prone skin behave.

Unfortunately for acne sufferers, once the hormones of pregnancy have reverted to their normal state, the acne condition may flare up. In some instances, this postpregnancy acne may be a woman's first experience with the condition.

· *Birth control pills.* It stands to reason that birth control pills can affect acne. How one is affected depends to some degree upon the kind of of pill prescribed. If you have acne-prone skin and are thinking of taking a birth control pill, make sure you discuss this with your doctor. Also if you are on the pill and get acne for the first time, the pill may be implicated.

· *Hormonal replacement therapy.* Any type of hormonal therapy or treatment can affect acne, sometimes making it worse; other times it makes it better. It all depends upon the type of hormone and the way the individual woman is responding to it.

Special Types of Acne

Adults can also be plagued by some special types of acne. Some of these are fairly unusual; still, they are worth mentioning.

Stress, Hormones, and Acne More and more, doctors are beginning to see a correlation between adult acne and stress. When you are under stress, or feeling fear or anxiety, your body sends out signals to your adrenal glands; they respond by activating your hormone levels. This sometimes means that there is an excess of androgens, setting off the chain by which the sebaceous glands are activated.

Cosmetic Acne Acne that is directly associated to the use of cosmetics that are themselves too oily for oily skin is unfortunately all too common. Cosmetics that can precipitate acne are known as comedegenic. Cosmetics that are designed with ingredients that are less likely to induce acne are known as noncomedegenic.

Drug Acne There are several drugs that have been known to trigger acne. These include: steroids, including cortisone; isonicotinic acid hydrazide (INH); synthetic adrenal-stimulating hormone (ACTH); diphenylhydantoin; danazol (often prescribed for women); and lithium carbonate, an anticonvulsant, including phenobarbital and Dilantin. Dr. James Fulton in his excellent book on acne also mentions marijuana as a drug that aggravates acne.

Iodine has also long been associated with acne, but most experts say that it is unlikely that there is enough iodine found in table salt to cause acne. However, vitamins as well as several prescribed medications sometimes contain enough iodine to precipitate an episode of acne.

Industrial Acne Some industrial compounds, including insoluble cutting oils, coal tar derivatives, and chlorinated hydrocarbons, may cause acne.

Tropical Acne Acne has been known to be triggered by tropical climates; this form of acne has been known to affect significant numbers of armed services personnel stationed in the tropics. Treatment often involves moving to a cooler climate.

Sun-related Acne This type of acne most often affects women in their twenties and thirties and appears to flare up after exposure to the sun.

Acne Mechanica Repetitive physical trauma is the causative factor in this form of acne, which can occur wherever a belt, strap, piece of clothing, or sports equipment has repeatedly rubbed against the skin. Some dermatologists also point out that repeated rubbing of the chin or forehead can lead to pimples.

Combination-Type Skin—What Is It?

Most of us have *combination-type skin*. But just because it's common doesn't mean that it's uncomplicated or easy to understand. Typically, the woman with combination-type skin has what is referred to as a T-zone (see the illustration on the next page). The skin in this T-zone area is oily, while the skin on the cheeks and other areas of the face surrounding the T-zone is dry.

Within this T-zone area, there may be sections that appear even oilier. The oiliest parts are usually found on the sides of the nose, particularly the corners where the nose meets the cheeks; the center of the chin; and the middle of the forehead. The pores in these oily sections will be large and may have a tendency to become plugged. Not everyone with combination-type skin gets pimples, but if you do, these are the trouble spots.

The skin on the rest of the face can be normal, or it can be dry. Normal or dry, the pores will be significantly smaller than those in the T-zone. If you are fortunate enough to have normal skin in the non-T-zone section, it will tend to be blemish-free and maintain a normal supply of both moisture and sebum. If the skin in this area is dry, it will often appear to be lacking in either moisture or oil.

Dermatologists sometimes see combination-type skin with a different and anomalous pattern, but T-zone is far and away the most likely.

The Most Extreme Combination-Type Skin—Pimples on the Nose and Chin and Dry Skin on the Cheeks If the skin on the side of your face is dry, but you are always waging war on pimples on your chin and the sides of your nose, you have an extreme version of combination-type skin. This can be a genuine problem, and if you are one of these women, the best thing you can do for your skin is to accept it, read up on both oily and dry skin, and treat each part accordingly.

Mild Combination-Type Skin Some lucky women have skin that is really almost normal, but under certain circumstances, they can develop comedones in their T-zones. Sometimes these women don't believe that they have combination skin and are not as careful as they should be about protecting the T-zone from excess oil.

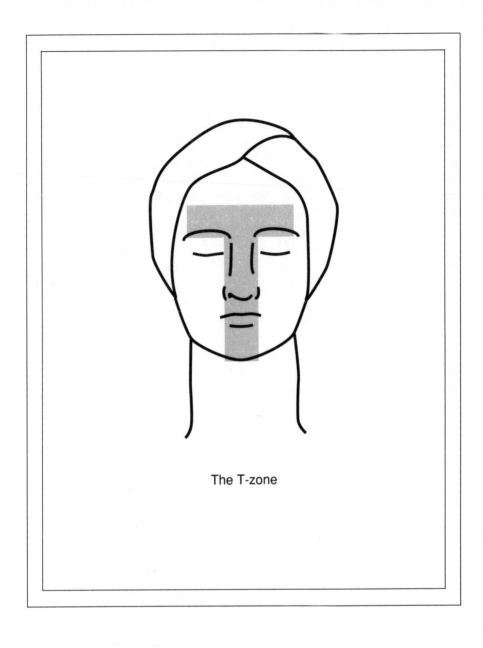

The T-zone

Normal Skin—What Is It?

Normal skin is skin in which all the parts are functioning properly. The oil glands are producing enough oil to keep the skin soft and smooth and protect it from moisture loss but not so much oil that the surface feels greasy or the pores get clogged.

Having normal skin does not mean that you never, ever, had a pimple. Mildly oily teenage skin usually turns out to be healthy normal skin.

If you are lucky enough to have normal skin, as an adult you should have few enlarged pores. They rarely get clogged and you're not troubled by pimples.

The thing to remember about normal skin is that even when you upset its naturally balanced state, its tendency is to return to a normal state. Normal skin, for example, may also respond to heavy oils by sprouting closed comedones. However, it will typically take longer for this to happen, and the flare-up will clear up faster than it does for oily skin. On the other hand, normal skin can also dry out from environmental factors and appear chapped, but the conditions have to be more extreme, and it is easier to bring your skin back to its normal moisture level.

THREE

Choosing and Using Skin Care Products

7

Products to Clean Your Face—Soaps, Cleansers, Toners, Masks, Scrubs

Cleaning one's face should be the least complicated skin care ritual, but this is not the case. While everyone in the skin care business agrees that clean, fresh skin is a good and desirable goal, no one seems to agree on how the average woman should go about cleaning her face or what sort of cleansing products she should use. This is particularly annoying because probably no other group of skin care products has as much potential for irritating the skin as those designed for cleansing. I think it is fair to say that most problems with mismanaged skin begin in the cleansing process.

Let's take a look at some of the products marketed to help you, and me, have clean skin: castile soaps and superfatted soaps, medicated soaps and gentle soaps, cream cleansers and foam cleansers, cleansing gels and cleansing bars, cleansing grains and nylon scrubs, cleansing milks and exfoliating toners. The list goes on and on and on, and it's mind-boggling. What is the right thing to do?

What do the experts advise? Some dermatologists say to stick to soap and water; others say that soap strips the body of natural oils. Alternatives to soap include cleansing creams and lotions, but there are dermatologists who warn us about the comedegenic risks involved in using oils or creams.

The skin care consumer receives the most confusing messages about facial cleansings whenever she walks through a cosmetics department. There she will probably be told that she needs everything: a cleansing cream for makeup removal; a toner or astringent to remove the cleansing cream; a scrub to remove the dead skin cells, etc. There are foaming cleansers, cleansing bars, regular cleansing lotions, mild cleansing lotions, and gentle cleansing lotions. What does all this mean?

How Should I Clean My Face? Let Me Count the Ways

Here are the five main ways in which you can clean your face:

Method 1: You can use a cleansing bar or liquid (either detergent or soap) and water to emulsify grease and dirt and wash them away. When you are finished, you rinse your face well with water. And your face is clean.

Method 2: You can use a product that is marketed or thought of as a cleansing cream. There are two types of products that are now marketed in the "cleansing cream" category. The first of these types is the old-fashioned "tissue off" cleansing cream. This is a product in which an oil such as mineral oil is used to remove grease, makeup, and dirt. Pond's Cleansing Cream is perhaps the best known. Over the years, some women have found that they get good results by designing their own cleansing creams, using an oil or grease such as baby oil or Crisco. When you are finished, your face is not totally clean because you are left with an oily film that should be removed.

The second type of "cleansing cream" includes products that aren't technically creams even though they may be loaded with emollients to soften the skin. These products, which are more soap or detergent than cream, are known as "rinse off" cleansers, and they are marketed in much the same way as cleansing creams so it is difficult to tell which you are buying. These products are sometimes called gels or foams.

Method 3: You can use toners and astringents, including an organic solvent such as alcohol, on your face to remove grease and dirt; they leave no residue and don't have to be rinsed off.

Method 4: You can use a scrub to clean surface dirt and exfoliate dead skin cells.

Method 5: You can use a mask to "deep clean" your pores and remove surface oils.

Before Talking About Soaps and Cleansers—Surfactant, a Word You Should Know

Before shopping for cleansing products, consumers should be aware of the term "surfactant." Surfactant simply means surface active agents. Surfactants are chemicals that reduce the surface tension of water, allowing it to spread out. Surfactants are sometimes irritating to the skin, but they are essential ingredients, necessary for removing dirt and oil. There are several categories of surfactants: anionic, nonionic, cationic, and amphoteric. Soaps are surfactants, and so are detergents. Some types of surfactants are milder than others. In cleansing preparations, surfactants are sometimes modified by the addition of emollients such as petrolatum or mineral oil.

Cleaning Your Face—Method 1: Talking About Soaps (and Detergents)

Until a few years ago, many dermatologists, tired of cosmetics hype, would treat all types of soap as equal and would often advise women to use whatever product was least expensive. Now, it has become apparent that all soaps are not alike and that some are definitely more irritating than others. Not only that, not all products marketed as soaps are really soaps—some are detergent bars. Some are also clearly marketed with specific skin types in mind, and several companies, such as Neutrogena, which sells its soap in dry, regular, acne, and baby formulas, now market similarly named products with slightly altered ingredients for different skin types.

Consumers are becoming more and more confused by all these different types of soaps. For one thing, some soaps list their ingredients on the label, while others do not. There is a reason for this. If you again read the FDA definition of a cosmetic, you will see that it expressly leaves out soap. A bar of soap is not considered a cosmetic and therefore the manufacturers don't have to tell the consumers what is in the product. There are many fewer restrictions about the type of ingredients, including what type of colors can be included in the product.

However, and this is the confusing part, a soap technically becomes a cosmetic if it is marketed as a cosmetic. Therefore, if the soap is marketed as cosmetic, that is, if the product is intended to beautify as well as to cleanse and a cosmetic claim such as "moisturization" or "exfoliation" is made, then the manufacturer is supposed to list the ingredients, and can use only permitted certified colors.

Because of this restriction, liquid soaps or "cream" soaps that are marketed as personal cleansing products are considered cosmetics, and manufacturers are supposed to follow FDA regulations and list ingredients.

If a soap is marketed as an anti-acne product, and it contains a legitimate ingredient in that category, then it is considered an over-the-counter drug, and the manufacturer has to fulfill all the regulations concerning over-the-counter drugs.

How Can the Consumer Tell Whether Her Soap Is a Soap, a Cosmetic, or a Drug? The fact is that she can't always tell the difference. If the soap expressly states that it is antimicrobial or anti-acne, then it is an over-the-counter drug, and the ingredients label should list the active ingredients. When it comes to plain old soaps and cosmetics, the consumer can't always tell the difference because some soap manufacturers list their ingredients even when they don't have to.

Shopping for a Soap—Some of the Choices

Soap has been around for a long time. According to the earliest sources, it was invented by the Mesopotamians about 2300 B.C. The value of soap is far more than cosmetic. In earlier cultures and in undeveloped areas where soap is at a premium, skin infections and other illnesses have been known to run rampant.

Today, of course, the concern for most skin care consumers is not which soap is going to do the best cleaning job, but which soap is going to not only clean, but also not strip oils, not upset the pH balance, not irritate, etc.

Old-fashioned Soap The basic old-fashioned soap is made by combining an alkali with a fat, often a vegetable oil, and water. Some of the old, traditional standbys such as Ivory soap fall into this category, but many of the products that we think of as soap are really synthetically produced detergents.

Detergent Soap Some consumers associate the word "detergent" with household cleansers and assume that a detergent soap is, by definition, going to be harsher than an ordinary soap. This is not the case. Although detergents are generally considered harsher than soaps, many companies modify their effect by adding extra emollients to the formula, making the cleansing product milder. One advantage to using detergents in cleansing bars is that it is easier to control the pH balance. Dove is an example of a familiar "soap" bar that is really a detergent bar.

pH-balanced Cleansing Product The pH scale measures whether something is acid, alkaline, or neutral. The pH value of 7.0 represents the neutral point. Anything above 7.0 is considered alkaline. Anything below 7.0 is considered acidic.

Sometimes you may see the phrase "acid mantle" used in reference to skin. The surface of the skin is covered by a film that is comprised of sebum (or oils), dead skin cells, and residue from the stratum corneum and perspiration. This film is what is meant by acid mantle; it typically has a pH that is mildly acidic. The pH of normal healthy skin usually averages between 4.5 and 6.5.

This pH represents a normal state. When we use a soap that is highly alkaline or an acid-based toner or astringent, we are briefly altering the pH level of the skin. A cleanser that is very alkaline will alter the pH, which in turn may cause the skin to feel dry or "tight." Healthy skin, however, quickly returns to its normal pH. Skin pH also changes, depending upon season, time of day, and location on the body.

Alkaline Cleaning Product An alkaline soap is one that has a pH that is above 7.0 and has an alkaline effect on the skin. This can be irritating, particularly for someone with dry skin.

Nonalkaline or pH-adjusted Cleansing Product Nonalkaline is what is usually meant when someone uses the term pH-balanced. Nonalkaline soaps will have a pH that is under 7.0 and should, theoretically, be less irritating. It would be wonderful if manufacturers were to list the pH of their soaps on the label, but unfortunately this doesn't happen very often. Most of the nonalkaline soaps are detergents.

Superfatted Cleansing Product Superfatted means what it sounds like: extra oils or fats such as lanolin, coconut oil, mineral oil, or cold cream are included in the soap formula, with the hope that these oils will replace some of those lost in the process of washing. Excess fatty acids are included in these formulas to insure that the pH is not exceedingly alkaline. An oily film that remains on your skin after washing can be a good thing if you have dry skin, and a bad thing if your skin is oily.

Glycerin Cleansing Product A glycerin soap is usually transparent and will often state that it is a glycerin soap. There are many popular soaps that include glycerin as an ingredient, including Basis and Neutrogena. Glycerin is known as a humectant.

Castile Cleansing Product Castile soap is often touted as being particularly pure, but in reality the basic difference between Castile soap and regular soap is that olive oil is used in the soap instead of another form of fat.

Medicated Cleansing Product The term medicated soap refers to a product that contains antibacterial ingredients. If a soap is medicated, it is a drug and, as such, is regulated by drug requirements. There are some medicated soaps that require a prescription. Most of the soaps recommended for acne are over-the-counter drugs.

Liquid Cleansing Product These are all over the place. Some are particularly designed for oily, acne-prone skin; others are specifically tailored for dry or sensitive skin. Many of these are modified detergents.

Deodorant Cleansing Products Deodorant soaps contain ingredients designed to fight body odor by killing off bacteria that live on the secretions from the apocrine sweat glands. These soaps are not recommended as facial cleansers. A few years ago most dermatologists suggested that you not use these soaps if you were planning to go out in the sun or be exposed to ultraviolet rays because they have been implicated in skin problems caused by photosensitivity. In a good number of instances, the manufacturers worked to resolve this problem and the problem ingredients have been removed. However, if you use a deodorant soap and plan to be in the sun, you might want to check with your dermatologist to see whether that particular soap has been given the green light for sun sensitivity.

As far as mildness is concerned, I know several women who swear by Dial, which is, of course, a deodorant soap, and, as a matter of fact, as you will see in the following section, when tested against several other well-known soaps for mildness, Dial certainly held its own.

Choosing a Mild Soap or Cleansing Product

Women, particularly those with dry or mature skin, are usually advised to choose a "mild" soap. Many women have asked me how they can determine which soaps are mild. Unfortunately, there have been very few comparison tests done on soaps. Some of you may have noticed, however, that many of the magazine and newspaper articles on skin care have recommended Dove soap. This is because of a study that was done in 1979 in which eighteen of the most popular soaps were tested and rated for irritancy by a group of researchers associated with the University of Pennsylvania. The soaps were rated for erythema, scaling, and fissuring and were assigned totals based on the results. They rated the eighteen soaps in the following order, starting with the mildest and ending with the harshest:

Dove, Aveenobar, Purpose, Dial, Alpha Keri, Fels Naphtha, Neutrogena, Ivory, Oilatum, Lowila, Jergens, Lubriderm, Cuticura, Basis, Irish Spring, Zest, Camay, and Lava.

Obviously, there is a whole variety of products that were not tested and that might rank right up there for mildness. Also, formulas for products do change, and some of these soaps may have new formulas that render them milder or harsher. It is only fair to point out that most of the soaps in the middle range were very close to each other in terms of totals.

Some Soap-Free Cleansers

Aveeno Cleansing Bar—a cleansing product that is unique because it includes colloidal oatmeal, along with a mild surfactant. It comes in medicated, oily, and dry-skin formulas. The dry-skin formula includes several emollients.

Cetaphil—a liquid cleanser often recommended for women with different skin types. It is completely free of lipids, or oils. Its primary ingredients are cetyl alcohol, stearyl alcohol, and sodium laurel sulfate, which is a detergent.

Dove—sold in most supermarkets. It is a popular detergent bar that tests have shown to be a mild and effective cleanser.

Keri Facial Cleanser—a liquid cleanser. Its ingredients include glycerin, propylene glycol, and squalane, along with such oil-absorbing ingredients as magnesium aluminum silicate.

Lowila—a bar product that includes emollients and softeners along with a detergent and boric acid.

pHisoderm Liquid—soap-free, unlike pHisoderm Gentle Cleansing Bar, and comes in dry, oily, and normal formulas.

Some pH-adjusted Soaps and Cleansers Washing the skin with harsh alkalis can alter the pH. Therefore some manufacturers have attempted to adjust the pH of their products in order to reduce this effect. Some of these products are:

Lowila Bar

Neutrogena Dry Skin Soap

Neutrogena (regular)

pHisoderm Liquid

Some Nondetergent Soaps The true-soap-versus-detergent argument has as many supporters as the pH-adjusted-detergent-versus-soap argument. If you want to stick to old-fashioned soap, here are some candidates:

Alpha Keri Moisturizing Soap

Basis, Glycerin Soap (Sensitive and Normal to Dry formulas)

Basis, Superfatted Soap

Cuticura Medicated Soap (mildly medicated soap that contains emollients)

Neutrogena Soap (Regular, Dry, and Baby Cleansing formulas)

Nivea Creme Soap

Oilatum

pHisoderm Gentle Cleansing Bar

Purpose Soap

Emollient Soaps Women with dry or mature skin often prefer using soaps or cleansing products that include moisturers. Here is a list:

Alpha Keri Moisturizing Soap

Basis, Superfatted Soap

Neutrogena Dry Skin Soap

Nivea Creme Soap

Oilatum

pHisoderm Gentle Cleansing Bar

Cleaning Your Face—Method 2: Talking About Cleansing Cream

Within the last few years, products that are marketed as cleansing creams have become even more complicated. Cleansing creams were originally designed as products that would clean skin without stripping the oils, and you may remember that a few years ago, the standard cosmetic product hype was that women who *really* cared about their skin didn't use soap.

Cleansing cream, which, by definition, leaves an oily film, was highly touted by most companies. Then the emphasis changed and people began talking about products that "didn't leave an oily film."

"Tissue Off"/"Rinse Off"

Now there are two separate and quite different types of products marketed as cleansing creams or lotions or sometimes foams. The first of these are the traditional cleansing creams, which typically contain a wax, mineral oil, water, and some form of detergent or soap. These are the old "tissue off" cleansing creams. Because cleansing creams were designed to clean your face without removing oil, they, of course, do leave an oily film.

"Tissue off" is one of the magic phrases used in determining whether the product is more cream than surfactant. If it says "tissue off," it means that you will be left with an oily film, which you are usually advised to remove with a toner or astringent.

"Rinse off" is the other phrase the consumer can look for in order to determine what kind of cleansing product she is buying. "Rinse off" means that the product is water soluble and probably has fewer oils. Even though "rinse off" products may look like lotions or creams and may be marketed in the same way as lotions or creams, they are usually primarily soaps or detergents, even though they may include oils for softening.

Cleansing "lotions" that are marketed for "oily" skin are often not lotions at all, but soaps or detergents. Cetaphil Lotion is an example that is found in drugstores. In department stores, products that are more soap than cream are sometimes called foams, or sometimes they are also called gels. The marketing usually doesn't help the consumer determine whether it is a soap or a cream. The only way to know for sure is to read the ingredients.

Now, to confuse the consumer totally, some companies sell products that they say can be "tissued off" or "rinsed off." In most instances, all this means is that the company is trying to get all parts of the cleansing cream market; usually this type of cleanser is a creamy lotion, which has the same sort of ingredients as the cleansing creams, but contains more water.

Examples of this type of product change can be found in several skin care lines. Good examples are two Lancôme products. The first is Douceur Demaquillante Nutrix, which is promoted as a "Gentle, *tissue off* cream cleanser for dry or sensitive skin." The first six ingredients are "mineral oil, water, isopropyl palmitate, propylene glycol, egg oil, vegetable oil." The second is Galatée, which is promoted as a "splash-or-tissue-away milky creme cleanser for every skin type." The first six ingredients in this product are "water, mineral oil, isopropyl myristate, propylene glycol, egg oil, vegetable oil."

If you read both lists of ingredients, you will note the primary difference is in the placement of the water. The "tissue off" Douceur Demaquillante Nutrix is a water-in-oil cleanser; it has more oil than water. The "splash-or-tissue-away" Galatée is an oil-in-water cleanser; it has more water than oil. But both products contain oil that ultimately should be removed from the skin. This is why salespeople for this type of product typically suggest using a toner or astringent after the cleansing cream or lotion.

Expensive "Tissue Off" Cleansing Creams— Some of the Negatives

Traditionally, cleansing creams have been promoted to women with dry skin. Obviously, women with oily or acne-prone skin don't want or need the extra emollients found in cleansing creams. However, the truth is that even though this type of product has been around for years, it is not an ideal choice for any woman, regardless of her skin type.

Here are some of the disadvantages for all skin types:

1. Cleansing creams leave an oily film on the face, and the cream must be removed by yet another product.

Women with oily skin absolutely don't want to run the unnecessary risk of leaving potentially comedegenic ingredients on their faces.

Women with dry skin sometimes make the mistake of thinking that they should leave the remains of their cleansing creams on the face. After all, they reason, if one has dry skin, what's wrong with adding oils. This is logical, but the typical cleansing cream also includes a soap-type ingredient such as sodium borate, which can be irritating for women with dry or sensitive skin.

2. Cleansing creams, even those targeted "for all skin types," may contain comedegenic ingredients that will irritate normal to oily skin types.

Some "Tissue Off" Cleansing Creams

Adrien Arpel Coconut Cleanser

Almay Deep Cleaning Cold Cream

Clinique Extremely Gentle Cleansing Cream

Dior Hydra Dior Cleansing Milk

Estée Lauder Tender Creme Cleanser

Lancôme Douceur Demaquillante Nutrix

La Prairie Cream Cleanser

Mary Kay Cleansing Cream Formula 1 (for dry to normal skin)

Noxzema Cold Cream

Pond's Deep Cleansing Cold Cream

Revlon's Moondrops Moisture Enriched Cream Cleanser

Shiseido Cleansing Cream

Some "Rinse Off" Cleansing Products The following products are technically not creams, but because they are sold as cosmetics rather than as soaps, the consumer often thinks of them as creams.

Clarins Gentle Foaming Cleanser

Lancôme Ablutia Gel Moussant

Mary Kay Cleanser Formula 3 (for oily skin)

Shiseido Cleansing Foam Concentrate (marketed for mature/dry skin)

Shiseido Facial Cleansing Foam (marketed for all skin types)

Some "Rinse Off" or "Tissue Off" Products These are the hybrids. Fundamentally, they are not completely water soluble, but they are less greasy than the ones marketed purely as "tissue off." In most instances, the manufacturers recommend following these products with a toner to thoroughly cleanse the skin.

Clarins Cleansing Milk with Alpine Herbs

Lancôme Galatée

Prescriptives Soothing Cream Cleanser

Other Popular Cleansing Products

Allercreme Combination Skin Cleanser

Almay Renewing Cleanser

Doak Formula 405 Soapless Cleansing Lotion

Estée Lauder Instant Rinse Off Cleanser

Estée Lauder Thorough Cleansing Gel

Ultima II Milky Facial Bath

Cleaning Your Face—Method 3: Talking About Toners, Clarifying Agents, Fresheners, Astringents, Etc.

All of these products have come to be known as toning lotions, and most skin care companies sell a variety of them, aimed at different needs. The term "toning lotion" is confusing to some women because they interpret the word "toning" to indicate that a toning lotion will somehow permanently firm up skin tissue. This is a logical assumption since the word is used in exercise class in referring to muscle development, but this is not what a toning lotion does. A toning lotion is simply another way of removing oil from your face, and it is traditionally used after cleansing cream for that reason. It is also sometimes recommended after soap and water cleaning in order to restore a mildly acid pH to the skin.

There are no guidelines to help the consumer distinguish among astringents, fresheners, clarifying agents, or toners. It's almost impossible to tell which you are buying unless you read the ingredients.

Here are some general guidelines:

Toning lotions can be broken down into two separate groups: Those that include alcohol as a primary ingredient; those that do not include alcohol.

In the toning lotions that include alcohol, the percentage of alcohol to water can vary a good deal. The higher the percentage of alcohol, the more drying the product. If you take a look at the ingredients of a toner that includes alcohol, you will often see the initials SD followed by a number. The initials SD stand for specially denatured. This indicates, among other things, that the alcohol is of the toxic nondrinkable variety.

Since alcohol is drying, it stands to reason that those products marketed for women with dry skin have little or no alcohol, while those intended for very oily skin have a higher percentage of alcohol.

The toning lotions that do not include alcohol typically include glycerin as well as a variety of plant extracts or sodium borate.

Astringents sometimes include alcohol as well as an ingredient, such as alum, which will make pores appear smaller, at least temporarily. This effect is created because alum, for example, will cause the pores to constrict.

When you see the term "pore lotion," it usually means that it specifically includes an ingredient to make pores appear smaller.

Clarifiers often contain an ingredient such as acetone, which acts to exfoliate the skin, thus taking away the top layer of dry epidermal cells and encouraging new cell action. This can produce shiny, clean-looking skin. Some companies, such as Clinique, make clarifying lotions in different strengths for different skin types.

Fresheners usually include alcohol, again in different strengths, depending upon the product, and their primary purpose is removing oil and thus "freshening" the skin.

Toning lotions often include a group of ingredients that are potentially irritating. These include camphor, menthol, sodium borate, eucalyptus oil, etc. These tend to give the skin a tingly sensation, which seems to reassure many women, particularly those with oily skin, that the product is "doing something."

Whenever you see the initials FD&C or D&C followed by a number and a color, you know the product contains a certified coal tar color. Although these colors are regularly included in everything from food to lipstick, it seems as though almost every year one or more of them are removed from products because they are proven to be carcinogenic in tests on lab animals. Some experts believe that many of these colors are comedegenic and/or irritants. They are not allowed in products formulated for use near the eyes.

Almost all astringents and toners have coal tar colors, and if this bothers you, keep in mind that many women use witch hazel, which is uncolored, either plain or diluted as a toner/astringent.

Some Toning Lotions That Include Alcohol

Adrien Arpel Herbal Astringent Lotion

Almay Moisture Balance Toner

Bonne Bell Ten-O-Six Lotion

Chanel Lotion Vivifiante

Clinique Clarifying Lotion #1, 2, 3

Contrôle de Lancôme

Lancôme Tonique Fraîcheur

La Prairie Cellular Purifying Lotion

Mary Kay Skin Freshener

Max Factor Skin Freshener

Sea Breeze

Some Toning Lotions That Do Not Include Alcohol

Adrien Arpel Lemon and Lime Freshener

Chanel Lotion Douce

Clarins Toning Lotion

Clinique Advanced Care Alcohol-Free Clarifier

Dior Hydra-Dior Lotion de Fraîcheur

Lancôme Tonique Douceur

La Prairie Cellular Refining Lotion

Prescriptives Skin Balancer

Other Popular Toning Products

Allercreme Astringent for Oily Skin

Allercreme Skin Freshener

Almay Oil Control Toner

Borghese Terme di Montecatini Stimulating Tonic

Dorothy Gray Activated Refining Lotion for Oily Skin

Elizabeth Arden Extra Control for Problem Skin Oil Clearing Astringent

Elizabeth Arden Visible Difference Refining Toner

Estée Lauder Full Strength Protection Tonic

Intelligent Skincare Detoxifying Lotion

Max Factor Moisture Rich Skin Freshener

Payot Lotion Aubelia

Ultima II Fresh Purifying Toner (Normal to Oily)

Ultima II Gentle Skin Balancing Lotion

Ultima II Lotion Refreshant (Normal to Dry)

Cleaning Your Face—Method 4: Talking About Scrubs and Exfoliation

---

When a skin care advertisement or a magazine article promotes a scrub-type product as one that aids in cell renewal, it sounds as though the product is doing something especially complicated. But it's not. Every time you use a washcloth on your face or a loofa on your back, you are using a scrub; you are exfoliating your skin and you are also encouraging cell renewal.

A scrub is any product that has an abrasive effect on your skin. A soft washcloth, for example, has a mild abrasive effect; a loofa has a strong abrasive effect.

Between your mildly abrasive washcloth and your more abrasive loofa are scads of moderately abrasive commercially manufactured skin care products as well as dozens of home prepared scrubs that can be whipped up in your kitchen. Commercially manufactured scrubs, which typically consist of abrasive particles that are suspended in a cleansing cream, are sometimes known by different names such as cleansing grains, washing grains, scrub cleansers, and sloughing cleansers.

Scrubs manufactured for dry skin will often include moisturizers as well as oils. Scrubs meant to be used on oily skin will sometimes include additional ingredients that help absorb oil. When you make your own homemade scrub, you may use only a handful of cornmeal or oatmeal, without any additional ingredients.

Another form of popular facial scrub is found in the special abrasive or cleansing sponges, such as the popular Buf-Puf.

There are many commonly used abrasive ingredients, including the well-known natural ones such as apricot seeds, almonds, walnuts, cornmeal, and oatmeal. Some synthetic ingredients include polyethylene powder, nylon powder, silica, and zirconium oxide.

The Good Things Scrubs Can Do for Your Skin

1. A scrub removes the dead cells on the top layer of the stratum corneum and, hence, encourages more rapid cell turnover.

Remember that the top layer of the epidermis, also known as the stratum corneum or horny layer, is made up of old, dried cells that have already died off. Removal of these worn-out old skin cells is sometimes called exfoliation or sloughing off because that's what happens when you use an abrasive scrub on the skin—the top layer of dried and dead skin cells is shed or exfoliated. This process encourages and stimulates the formation of new skin cells in the basal layer, or lowest layer, of the epidermis, which is where new epidermal cells are formed.

2. A scrub will massage the skin and improve circulation.

Circulation is another function that decreases with age. Most of us have noticed that as we age, our skin becomes paler. Massaging of the skin with a scrub ideally improves color and gives the skin a rosy glow.

3. A scrub removes excess oil from the skin.

This is a very good thing to do if you have oily skin. One of the unpleasant features of oily skin is that the oils form a bond around the top layer of skin cells, and they are not as easily exfoliated as are dry skin cells. Removing this top oily layer makes the skin look smoother, finer, and clearer. Removing excess oil often also reduces the incidence of pimples.

If you have dry skin and don't have enough oil, you want to get rid of the dead skin cells without losing too much oil. You can do this by using a scrub in which the abrasive particles are suspended in an oil, and thus put back some of the oil that is removed.

4. To clean the skin and pores.

We all know that clean skin looks brighter and healthier. Well, nothing seems to beat a scrub for getting the skin squeaky clean and removing the glop from clogged pores.

5. To polish and soften the skin.

Smooth, soft skin is fun to touch. Consumers tend to forget about polishing the skin to get an extra smooth and soft feel as well as a shiny, glowing look.

What a Scrub Will Not Do

A scrub will not get rid of blemishes, blackheads, whiteheads, or pimples. It is not intended as a means of scrubbing away pimples or skin problems. In fact, a scrub *should not* be used on pimples or skin that is broken.

The best thing about scrubs is that some of the best are those you make yourself for pennies, using products such as oatmeal, or cornmeal, or finely powdered almonds. The more expensive department store cosmetic scrub products typically combine creams and oils with the abrasive ingredient, but by and large these creams are not essential to the way the scrub works. Some companies don't manufacture scrubs, but they do market facial cleansing brushes, which they recommend using with their cleansing products. These essentially have the same effect as the traditional scrubs.

Scrubs That Do Not Include Creams or Oils

cornmeal

oatmeal

Adrien Arpel Sea Kelp Cleanser

Buf-Puf (gentle and regular)

Lancôme La Brosse Douceur D'Eau (gentle cleansing brush)

Shiseido Facial Cleansing Brush

Scrubs That Do Include Creams or Oils

Adrien Arpel Honey and Almond Scrub

Clinique 7-Day Scrub Cream

Prescriptives Skin Refiner

Other Popular Scrub Products

Allercreme Scrub Masque

Almay Oil Complexion Scrub

Clinique Exfoliating Scrub

Elizabeth Arden Visible Difference Gentle Scrub Creme

Estée Lauder Gentle Action Skin Polisher

Estée Lauder Solid Milk Cleansing Grains

Lancôme Exfoliance Delicate Facial Buff

Ultima II Deep Pore Scrub Masque

Cleansing Your Face—Method 5: Talking About Masks

Masks are among the oldest form of cleansing products. Typically, the promotional material for cleansing masks will use terms such as "deep cleans." Cleansing masks are but another way to remove excess oil and dirt, along with dead skin cells. There are, of course, masks that are sold as moisturizing agents. These will usually be promoted with language such as "nourishing" or "moisturizing."

Cleansing masks are broken down into two categories: wash offs and peel offs. Wash-off masks are traditionally made from some form of clay or "mud." When you apply the clay product to your face, the water evaporates and the clay hardens; as it does so, it lifts up excess oil and dirt. Peel-off masks are usually made with ingredients such as vinyl acetate or polyvinyl alcohol. The product is applied as a film to the face and left to dry. When it is dry, it forms a sheet of sheer vinyl, which the consumer can peel away. As she does so, the vinyl layer lifts away dirt and dead skin cells.

Facial Masks (Rinse Off)

Kiehl's Rare-Earth Masque

Mudd Mask

Shiseido Facial Masque (clay rinse off)

Facial Masks (Peel Off)

Bonne Bell Orange Peel Masque

Revlon Moon Drops Honey Masque (peel off)

Shiseido Facial Masque (peel off)

Other Popular Masques

Almay Deep Pore Cleansing Mask

Coty Sweet Earth Masks (Mud and Peel Away)

Estée Lauder Almond Clay Mask

Orlane Masks

Payot Authentique Masque Creme

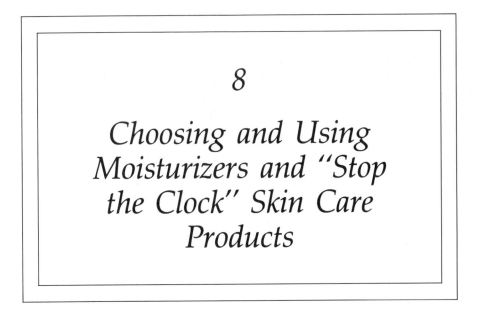

8

Choosing and Using Moisturizers and "Stop the Clock" Skin Care Products

In grandma's day, there were two basic kinds of face cream—cold cream and vanishing cream. Cold cream was the kind you put on at night, or if no one was looking, because all cold creams were sticky, gooey, and greasy. Vanishing creams were something women could use during the day because they were less greasy and hence "vanished." I remember those vanishing creams from my childhood. It seems to me that glycerin was a major ingredient. Also, while yesteryear's products didn't leave a greasy film, they also didn't produce a youthful sheen. As a matter of fact, if memory serves me right, they sort of lay there on the top of the skin, reflecting a dull, matte finish.

Those vanishing creams are the ancestors of today's ultrasophisticated moisturizers. Today's moisturizers aren't greasy, and they aren't dull-looking. Women love them because they make their skin look terrific. Cosmetics companies love them because the women who love them spend well over a billion dollars a year buying them—moisturizers account for approximately 60 percent of the cosmetic skin care business.

Moisturizers improve the skin's appearance because they make it appear and feel softer and smoother. They do this by bringing moisture, or water, into the epidermis. This moisture causes the epidermal skin cells to plump up.

Remember, that as skin ages, skin cells lose a part of their capacity to retain moisture. Also remember that the stratum corneum, or top layer of skin, is made up of skin cells that have become flattened and dry. However, these cells have the capacity to absorb water or moisture that is placed on the surface of the skin. When these cells have absorbed a sufficient amount of moisture, they swell up and press closer to each other. This plumping process smooths the skin's surface and makes surface lines temporarily disappear; some wrinkles therefore appear to have less depth.

If you rinse your face with water, the cells will promptly start to soak up moisture. But within a very short period of time, this water will evaporate, and the cells will be flat and dry-looking again. Simply adding water to the skin will not resolve the dry skin problem. You also have to replace the skin's natural oils with another oily or occlusive substance to keep the water from evaporating into the atmosphere. That's how moisturizing creams work. They introduce the moisture or water to the cells, but they also include an oil, known as an occlusive, which spreads over the surface of the skin and retards transepidermal water loss.

If you want to do this for yourself while spending only pennies, you could splash your face with cool water for about five minutes and then quickly spread any greasy substance such as petrolatum or Crisco on your skin. The cells would fill up with water and plump up, and the greasy film would reduce evaporation or water loss. It's simple.

However, the typical skin care consumer doesn't want to walk around with grease on her face. She wants to look terrific, which is why she is taking care of her skin. An oily face doesn't look terrific. Besides, you can't apply makeup on slippery skin.

The cosmetics industry is acutely aware of the consumer's aversion to the greasy look, and it is prepared to provide her with dozens of alternatives, which will not cost pennies. They will cost dollars. Some cost many dollars. These moisturizers are touted in advertisements and promotions, many of which talk about complicated new ingredients. All of this tends to lead the consumer to believe that these new products are more effective moisturizers than inexpensive old standbys such as petrolatum. In reality, this is not necessarily the case.

Greasy/Nongreasy—What's the Difference?

The old-fashioned face creams were known as water-in-oil substances. The products that the skin care companies refer to as moisturizers are known as oil-in-water substances. They are sometimes also called lotions. If you look at the ingredients label of just about any moisturizer or lotion, you will see that water is the first ingredient listed. The second ingredient is usually the emollient or oil. Often it will be mineral oil or petrolatum. In other words, moisturizers have more water than oil. Hence the term oil-in-water. That's why they are less greasy than their predecessors. Some products, which are often called skin oils, are water-in-oil substances. For example, Nivea Skin Oil is a water-in-oil product, and if you look at the ingredients you will see that mineral oil is the first ingredient listed, and water is the second. These water-in-oil products feel oilier and greasier.

Moisturizers with a lot of oil are thicker than those with only a little. These are known as heavy moisturizers. Moisturizers that have more water feel watery. These are known as light moisturizers. Most of the new moisturizers, both the day and night variety, are designed to feel fairly light, but women still tend to think of a daytime moisturizer as being lighter than a nighttime product.

Some Frequently Used Moisturizer Ingredients and What They Do

Water

Water is the first and most important ingredient in a moisturizer. Water is the substance that brings the moisture to your skin cells.

Emollients

The emollient is typically the second ingredient in a moisturizer. An emollient is a substance that forms an occlusive barrier on the skin through which water cannot pass. The terms "emollient" and "occlusive" are often used synonymously. When you put an emollient on your skin, the moisture in your skin, and the water in the moisturizing product, cannot be easily lost into the environment because emollients prevent moisture loss, from evaporation, from the surface of your skin. The most commonly used emollients are petrolatum, lanolin, mineral oil, and the silicones.

Petrolatum Most dermatologists will tell you that petrolatum is far and away the most effective emollient and moisturizer. Nothing else comes close in terms of forming a protective shield on the surface of your skin.

Petrolatum has been listed in the *United States Pharmacopoeia* since 1880. It was originally introduced to the cosmetics industry by Robert A. Chesebrough, who called it Vaseline, which is now a trademark of Chesebrough-Pond's.

Several studies have been done that point out the effectiveness of petrolatum as a moisturizer. A ten-year dermatological study by the researchers at the University of Pennsylvania studied different moisturizers on women who had very dry skin on their legs. The women were asked to use a variety of occlusives on their legs for fourteen days, and then the results were checked.

The winner: Petrolatum was the most effective; its benefits lasted for about two weeks after the final application.

Women tend to associate petrolatum with a sticky, greasy feel, but new formulations are being introduced that contain different concentrations, and many of the newer products that derive their emolliency from petrolatum do not feel greasy.

Petrolatum has another plus in that it is rarely mentioned as an allergen or a sensitizer.

Lanolin and Lanolin Derivatives After petrolatum, lanolin was cited as the second most effective emollient tested, and it is included in a variety of both expensive and inexpensive skin care products designed for dry skin. If you have dry skin and are not sensitive to lanolin, it is a terrific ingredient because lanolin, which is extracted from sheep wool, is very close in composition to sebum, the oil that is secreted naturally by your sebaceous glands. As an emollient, it is extremely effective in preventing water loss from the skin, and it is also effective as a skin softener.

Unfortunately, lanolin is frequently cited as a potential sensitizer or allergen. As to whether or not lanolin is comedegenic, there seems to be some disagreement. Some experts rank lanolin and its derivatives as extremely comedegenic. Others do not. If I had acne or acne-prone oily skin, I think I would opt for a better-safe-than-sorry approach. It makes sense that if lanolin is so close in composition to sebum then, like sebum, it might be comedegenic.

The different forms of lanolin are: acetylated lanolin, acetylated lanolin alcohol, lanolin, lanolin acid, lanolin alcohol, lanolin oil.

Mineral Oil Mineral oil, which is included as an emollient in approximately 4,000 products, is the most common cosmetic and skin care ingredient. It is found in just about everything from baby oil to foundation makeup. Over the years, I have met a few women who told me that they had allergic reactions to mineral oil, but it is rarely considered a sensitizer, and most of us tolerate it extremely well. Because it is an oil, it is not normally included in products for acne-prone skin, but many dermatologists feel that it is not even all that comedegenic.

Although mineral oil is probably not as effective as petrolatum or lanolin in preventing moisture loss from the skin, it is also not as "sticky" as petrolatum nor as much of a sensitizer as lanolin.

Humectants

After emollients, humectants are the next most popular category of moisturizing ingredients. Typically, most moisturizers contain both a humectant and an emollient.

Humectants are included in a variety of day and night moisturizers because they have a special moisturizing ability. A humectant is an ingredient that can absorb moisture from the environment. What this actually means is that if you put on your skin a moisturizer that includes a humectant, it can attract and absorb moisture from the air around you. Because this moisture from the environment is then on your skin, it is available to the stratum corneum. Isn't that efficient?

The most common humectants are propylene glycol and glycerin, and if you look at most moisturizers, you will see that one of these humectants is included.

For reasons too complicated for me to understand, undiluted glycerin can sometimes have a dehydrating effect on the skin, and for these reasons it is not considered an effective moisturizer unless it is diluted in the 20 to 45 percent concentration range.

The other problem with humectants, including propylene glycol and glycerin, is that although they are most effective when you are in areas with high humidity, if you are going to be in an extremely low humidity atmosphere, such as in an airplane, or even a very dry room, they can actually take moisture from your skin. Here's why: Humectants are on the search for moisture that can be absorbed from the environment. If the environment is so drying that there is no moisture to be had, they will get it from the next best source—your skin. When this happens, the ingredient, which is supposed to help your skin retain moisture, instead does the opposite.

Propylene glycol, which is included in many products, is sometimes cited as an allergen, but some experts believe that, typically, a woman will become sensitive to the ingredient only when she is in a very low humidity environment, in which case the propylene glycol can become irritating.

Natural Moisturizing Factor (NMF)

Natural moisturizing factor, or NMF, is a term we see quite often in magazine articles on skin care. What the term means is quite vague and open to a certain amount of controversy. Basically, the term refers to a group of ingredients that are found naturally in the body and that seem to have the capacity to bind or hold water to the skin. Probably the best-known components of the NMF are urea and lactic acid.

Urea is used in moisturizers because of its water-binding capacity. It is also a very effective skin softener and is very helpful in treating skin that is flaky and cracking. Another advantage is that it is not greasy.

Lactic acid has a solid history as a moisturizing and softening agent for dry skin. In higher concentrations, some dermatologists use lactic acid as an exfoliating agent.

Other NMFs include collagen, hyaluronic acid, mucopolysaccharides, NaPCA (sodium pyrrolidone carboxylate), which is marketed as Ajidew, and hydroxy acids such as lactic acid.

Other Popular Moisturizing Agents

Aloe   Aloe, which is also called aloe vera, may be the most popular of the so-called natural ingredients. The name aloe comes from the Arabic, *alloeh,* or the Hebrew, *halal,* both of which indicate that aloe is a bitter, shiny substance.

The aloe plant produces two different types of substances that we use. One, a bitter reddish-yellow juice, is sometimes used as a laxative and, when dry, is the form of aloe recognized in the *United States Pharmacopoeia.*

The second aloe substance, which is also sometimes called juice, looks more like colorless gelatin. It is this gel that is most commonly included in skin care products.

Why is aloe used in so many skin care products? Chemical analysis of aloe has shown the presence of mucopolysaccharides, which is a natural moisturizing factor, enzymes such as catalase and cellulase, minerals such as calcium, aluminum, iron, zinc, magnesium, potassium, and sodium, as well as amino acids. Aloe also has a pH that is in the same range as normal skin.

Because it is primarily a mucopolysaccharide, aloe is seen as a moisturizing agent. It is infrequently cited as an allergen.

Here are some of the claims that have been made for aloe.

· Undiluted aloe is helpful in treating or preventing hyperpigmentation, known as liver spots.
· Lab animals whose skins were treated with aloe on a daily basis for up to four months showed an increase in the soluble collagen content of the skin.
· Aloe improves the way skin looks by improving hydration.
· Aloe may have an analgesic effect on inflammation, burns, and minor skin irritations.

Jojoba Oil Like aloe, jojoba is considered a natural ingredient. Jojoba oil comes from the seeds of a bush that is native to the American Southwest. Jojoba is often used as a moisturizing agent, and some of its proponents suggest that it is a particularly valuable ingredient because it doesn't appear to be a comedegenic and may even serve a useful function in products designed for oily skin.

Triglycerides A great many of the familiar sounding oils are triglycerides including: apricot kernel oil, avocado oil, caprylic/capric triglycerides, castor oil, cocoa butter, coconut oil, corn oil, grape seed oil, soybean oil, mink oil, olive oil, sesame oil, shea butter, sweet almond oil, wheat germ oil, and peach kernel oil.

Allantoin Allantoin is probably not as effective as urea as a skin softener, but it is included in many skin care products because of its anti-irritant and soothing qualities. It would appear that allantoin inhibits allergic-type responses and may weaken the effects of some skin sensitizers. For this reason, allantoin is often used in products for women with sensitive skin.

Getting Expensive—Moisturizers That Claim Upscale Ingredients

Once upon a time all a moisturizer was expected to do was to relieve dry skin. The new moisturizing products sold at department store cosmetics counters are making fancier claims. Many of the cosmetics companies are claiming that their products are to be taken seriously in the wrinkle war. To reinforce their claims, many of the new moisturizers have ultrasophisticated packaging; La Prairie's caviar-like globes that look like small pearls is just one of the new packaging innovations.

But the packaging is not all that's new. If you read the ads for products like Lauder's Night Repair or Prescriptive's Line Preventor or Dior's Capture or Lancôme's Niosôme, you can't help but notice that these products claim a whole group of ingredients that sound more sophisticated than plain old-fashioned petrolatum or mineral oil. Here are some of them:

Epidermal Lipids The epidermis naturally contains a whole range of lipids, or oils, including cholesterol, glycolipids, phospholipids, and free fatty acids. All of these lipids are natural moisturizers and as such are included in many skin care products.

Collagen Collagen, which is the major structural protein in the human dermis, starts to change when we get older. Like everything else, collagen loses its bounce. As our bodies' natural supplies of collagen age, our skin begins to sag. The rationale for including collagen in skin care products is that external application will be able to impart to aging skin some of the characteristics of young skin. However, applying collagen to the surface of the skin will not do that. It can't, because the collagen molecule is much too large to be absorbed by the epidermis, and it certainly can't penetrate into the dermis itself.

However, after saying that, it's important for the consumer to realize that collagen is still an excellent ingredient because it is a very efficient moisturizing agent and it helps hold water in your skin.

Collagen is found in many popular skin care products. Perhaps the best known is Ultima's ProCollagen.

Mucopolysaccharides Mucopolysaccharide is the name given to certain substances that, like collagen and elastin, are found in the human dermis. Hyaluronic acid is the principal mucopolysaccharide. Hyaluronic acid is a favorite skin care ingredient because it is a good moisturizer. There is another reason given for including it in moisturizers: When your skin is exposed to ultraviolet rays, the natural amount of hyaluronic acid in your skin decreases. The rationale is that by applying hyaluronic acid to your skin, you will somehow be able to replace what was lost from your dermis. Unfortunately, it doesn't work that way because hyaluronic acid cannot be externally absorbed into the dermis. Other mucopolysaccharides include chondroitin sulfates.

Some well-known skin care products that contain hyaluronic acid include Estée Lauder's Night Repair and Shiseido's B.H.–24.

Alpha Hydroxy Acids Alpha hydroxy acids are naturally occurring substances found in many fruits and vegetables, including malic acid (apple juice), citric acid (citrus fruit), tartaric acid (wine), and lactic acid (sour milk). Most cosmetic products do not include adequate amounts of alpha hydroxy acids to affect the skin, but there is some new research being done that combines the acids with other drugs; this research may hold promise for drug-type ingredients that can be used to smooth wrinkles.

Thymus Extracts The FDA says nonsense, but some skin care companies claim that extracts of animal thymus glands can stimulate cell renewal, and there have actually been some studies indicating that thymus extracts might indeed have a beneficial effect on the skin.

Liposomes and Niosomes These are not really ingredients. They are what is known as "delivery systems." They are very, very tiny, hollow lipid spheres. Imagine a small balloon made of oil and shrunk beyond what the human eye can see. Chemistry has made it possible to do just that. Some skin companies say that these little spheres can penetrate the surface of the skin and "deliver" the ingredients inside. Inside these hollow spheres, some companies have placed ingredients, which they say will penetrate the skin because they are "delivered" by the lipid spheres.

Dior's Capture features liposomes that contain, among other things, thymus extracts.

Lancôme's Niosôme features niosomes that contain, among other things, the natural moisturizing factor known as NaPCA.

The FDA and many dermatologists sincerely question whether these "delivery systems" can deliver the goods, but in the meantime many women love the products.

Vitamins In recent years, vitamins, particularly the antioxidants, A, C, and E, have started to get a great deal more play in skin care promotions.

Vitamin A (retinol) has received a great deal of publicity because it is in the same family as the drug Retin-A. If you look at skin care promotions, you will see that more and more companies are including forms of this vitamin in their products. Vitamin A (retinol) does not have the same results as Retin-A.

Vitamin E (tocopherol) has a long history of use and although many of its quoted successes are anecdotal, a great many people say they use it on bruises, cuts, and skin irritations and sometimes on their animals. Many who do so swear by vitamin E. But to date, there is little research that clearly shows its effectiveness except as a moisturizing agent. Because new research is being done, this situation may change and there may soon be something more definitive. Some experts suggest that di-alpha-tocopherol acetate can be an effective agent in preventing irritation and is helpful in reducing the negative effects of ultraviolet light.

Vitamin C (ascorbic acid or vitamin C derivative ascorbyl palmitate) is an essential vitamin that serves many functions within the body. Among these, the vitamin in combination with bioflavonoids helps prevent collagen breakdown. Several skin care products, including Avon's

Collagen Booster, refer to the way in which vitamin C and collagen interact. And they do. Whether this interaction can take place by applying vitamin C on the skin is another matter; most experts believe that it cannot.

Sometimes these vitamins are used in different forms or for other purposes. An example is di-alpha-tocopherol nicotinate, which works via vasodilation. All that means is that some experiments have been done in which di-alpha-tocopherol nicotinate is applied to the skin with the hope of improving microcirculation.

Understanding the Ingredients/Understanding the New Claims

There is a lot of technical language being used to promote some of the newer skin care products. In some instances, however, these words are attached to the same old ingredients. Here are some of the more common skin care claims, along with what they mean and some of the ingredients most likely to be included in the product.

"Cell Renewal" A cell renewal claim is most likely to be made for a product that in some way exfoliates the skin or includes an ingredient that creates that effect. This exfoliation process can be induced by something as simple as a scrub, such as a Buf-Puf, or any product that includes an ingredient that irritates the skin slightly, thus speeding up cell renewal. Some typical ingredients include soap, detergents, polyethylene, ground fruit pit materials such as apricot kernels, and fruit acids.

Cell renewal is a major buzz word in the skin care business, but although it makes the skin look better, it doesn't create younger skin. Although you may end up with new cells in the epidermis, you still have the same dermis, which is why you still have the same old wrinkles.

"Microcirculation" As we get older, circulation is diminished. This is why the skin gets whiter and paler as we grow older. Anything that brings blood to the surface of the skin increases microcirculation. Massaging the skin increases microcirculation. So does using a scrub product on

the skin. Ingredients that increase microcirculation include witch hazel, some plant extracts, and botanicals.

"Temporary Wrinkle Smoothing" Temporary means temporary, but it is still nice every now and then to be able to get a smoother look. Some ingredients include sodium silicate, bovine serum albumin, and human placental protein.

"Repair Intercellular Network"/"Repair Damage Done to Skin by Ultraviolet Light"/"Night Repair" Chondroitin sulfate, hyaluronic acid, and other mucopolysaccharides form part of the intercellular network of the dermis, and they are damaged by ultraviolet light. Claims of this nature usually indicate that the product contains one or more of these ingredients. However, it has not been shown that external application of these ingredients will affect the dermis. But they are all good moisturizing agents.

"Environment Creams"/"Airplane Creams" Anyone who has been in an airplane for more than a couple of hours knows that the air within the plane is extraordinarily dry. This happens because at high altitudes the air is very cold and it must be heated before it can be circulated in the cabin. This heating process removes moisture from the air.

Because so many flight attendants complained of dry skin, several manufacturers including Estée Lauder began to make creams that addressed the issue of extremely dry air. These dry conditions also occur environmentally in desert areas in the American Southwest.

Creams formulated for low humidity environments should be high in water and emollients. They may also contain a silicone such as dimethicone or cyclomethicone because they will provide a seal on the skin. Humectants such as propylene glycol and glycerin are not ideal choices.

"Free Radical Protection" and the Role of Natural Antioxidants
If you walk around cosmetics counters these days, chances are you're going to hear a lot about the dangers of the free radical and how and why using a particular moisturizer or sunscreen will protect you.

The concept of the free radical, which is sometimes discussed as an unpaired electron, is very complicated. I certainly don't understand it, and about the only thing I can say with any degree of certainty is that the men and women who are selling skin care products seem to understand it even less. The last time I was at a cosmetics counter, a saleswoman told me that the moisturizer she was selling was "so high in free radical formulations that it wipes the ultraviolet rays right off your face."

Meaningless scientific babble notwithstanding, it is now acknowledged by experts in many fields, including medicine and biology, that the free radical is directly implicated in the aging process and in disease. You really can't get away from free radicals. They are caused by pollution, ultraviolet light, harsh environmental conditions, including impaired ozone and radiation, some foods, as well as living in general. Some theories say that free radicals destroy some cells and in the process create wrinkles.

It has been discovered that antioxidants help prevent free radical damage, and there are some scientists who are willing to consider the possibility that ingesting antioxidants in the form of vitamins can limit the damage because antioxidants really do seek out and destroy free radicals. Some well-known antioxidants include vitamin E (tocopherol), beta-carotene (a vitamin A precursor found in carrots and other vegetables), vitamin C (ascorbic acid), bioflavonoids, and superoxide dismutase.

Several of the skin care companies, including Avon, Estée Lauder, Shiseido, etc., have begun to include antioxidants in their skin care products.

However, some experts question whether applying antioxidants topically can have the desired preventive effect. Others feel that antioxidants are a requirement for any product that is attempting to reduce wrinkles or aid in wrinkle control.

Estée Lauder's Line Preventor has been promoted as a "free radical scavenger," and the promotion for Revlon's Age Less face capsules indicates that the product will block free radical formation.

The director of the FDA's cosmetics division has been quoted as saying that there is no proof that free radicals cause wrinkles and there is no reason to believe that applying antioxidants on the skin will have any effect on skin cells. Once again, the FDA's attitude seems to be that if all these antioxidants were able to alter or change skin cells, then the skin care companies should have the products tested as drugs.

In the meantime, here is a list of some of the more familiar antioxidant and vitamin ingredients that consumers are likely to find in their skin creams. Remember that, when used as cosmetic ingredients, vitamins A, E, C, etc., are supposed to be listed by their technical names.

"Anti-Aging"/"Prevents Premature Aging"/"Protection from Ultraviolet Light" The only products that are supposed to make an anti-aging claim are those that contain an over-the-counter sunscreen ingredient. These approved sunscreen ingredients do prevent premature aging caused by solar damage, and they do protect from ultraviolet light.

"Nonocclusive or Oil-Free Moisturizing" Moisturizers formulated for women with oily skin typically will not contain an occlusive, or emollient. Instead, these products can include propylene glycol, hyaluronic acid, lactic acid, collagen, and NMF ingredients.

Within the last ten years, increasingly sophisticated research has created a whole new generation of skin care ingredients and skin care products. One can clearly see how these new ingredients have created a completely new set of claims for the products in which they are included. Some of these products are quite expensive. It can cost $60 or more for a two-ounce jar of moisturizer. Compared to $6 for eight ounces of a petrolatum-based moisturizer, it is no wonder the consumer is beginning to ask, "Are these products really worth all this money?" What the consumer has to decide is whether these new skin care products do everything the ads promise they will and whether they are more efficient than the less expensive moisturizers found on drugstore shelves.

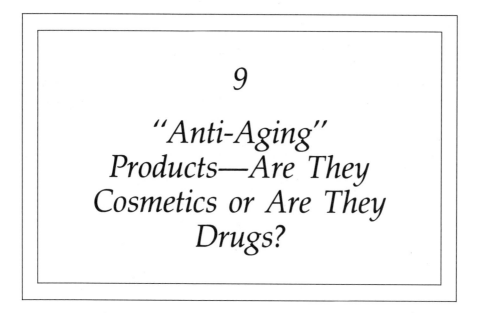

9

"Anti-Aging" Products—Are They Cosmetics or Are They Drugs?

Do Skin Care Products Do Everything the Ads Promise They Will?

If I knew for sure that these products worked, I would be the first person in the stores, and hang the expense, but I'm not sure which, if any, do work, and I remember what Charles Revson said about "hope in a bottle." I don't want to squander my money on hope.
—LAURA M., THIRTY-EIGHT-YEAR-OLD CONSUMER

I think Laura's reaction is typical. Just about every woman over thirty has read ads or seen promotional literature that has made her wonder whether she should rush out and invest in one of the newer products. As a matter of fact, the two questions I'm most often asked are, "Do skin care products really work" and "Do skin care products do everything the ads promise they will?"

Do most of you remember when skin care products first became big business? It was the late 1960s, and at that time the claims surrounding skin care products tended to restrict themselves to skin moisturization, with an occasional cleansing product thrown in. Typical ads talked about "smoother" and "suppler" skin. "Hypoallergenic" and "natural" were about as complicated as anyone got.

However, if you have browsed through any of the magazines within the last few years, you couldn't help noticing the skin care ads and the way in which so many companies started referring to their products as "skin treatment." The industry seemed to decide that the scientific approach was definitely the way to go. Every new product that was being launched was accompanied by reams of scientific research, complete with diagrams and photographs illustrating supposedly documented changes in moisturization or the depth of individual wrinkles. And, as the promotional literature became more and more "scientific," the claims became more and more daring in terms of what was promised to the skin care consumer.

The problem is that no one seems to be able to verify whether any, or all, of these products really do live up to all of their scientific jargon. In short, do they work? Before we can decide whether these products deliver, as promised, I think we have to look at some of the actual words that have been used by cosmetics companies in their advertising and labeling and see what it is that they are really saying.

Here are some examples of claims used in advertisements or promotional material in the mid-1980s:

Biotherm, a skin care line owned by Cosmair

> For Biotherm Actif Nuit Nighttime Stress Reducer: "Counteracts the signs of premature aging caused by tension and stress. . . . Increases skin's natural powers of regeneration."

> For Biotherm Special Rides Anti-Wrinkle Cream: "Problem: Is there a way to visibly diminish my wrinkles? Solution: BIOTHERM. To protect against the ravages of time."

Estée Lauder

> For Estée Lauder Night Repair, a product that calls itself a "cellular Recovery Complex": ". . . contains a complex of natural ingredients that supplements your own skin's repair mechanisms . . . beauty breakthrough that changed the science of skin care to skin repair."

Lancôme

> For Lancôme Niosôme Système Anti-Age Daytime Skin Treatment: ". . . recreate the structure of a young skin . . . helps to rebuild the intercellular network of your skin."

Avon

For BioAdvance Beauty Recovery System: ". . . actually helps reverse many signs of facial aging . . . in just six weeks."

For Avon Collagen Booster Line Controlling Lotion: ". . . actually helps prevent many of the visible signs of aging . . . helps supplement the natural production of fresh young collagen."

Jacqueline Cochran's La Prairie

For La Prairie Cellular Restorative Complex: ". . . new cells at the surface are plumper and younger . . . most important, the skin itself now has improved quality."

Glycel, a skin care line owned by Alfin Fragrances

Best known as the company that introduced glycosphingolipids (GSL) in the Glycel GSL Cellular Line, they marketed Glycel GSL Cellular Treatment Activator, GSL Cellular Anti-Aging Creme, and GSL Cellular Night Creme. Some of the language they used in advertising and labeling included: "Isolated by Dr. Christiaan Barnard, world-renowned heart surgeon, and a team of Swiss cell biologists. Dr. Barnard has discovered that when aging skin is supplied with GSL, it can function as if it were young again. . . ."

Princess Marcella Borghese

For Hydro-Minerali Skin Revitalizing Extract: ". . . help restore skin's vibrancy, resiliency, and luminosity. . . . Minerals . . . are essential to every cell's life-giving metabolic processes, including oxygenation and the removal of toxins."

Do the Ads Mean What They Say or Do They Seem to Say Something They Don't Mean?

That's sort of a funny, convoluted question, but anyone who has ever tried to dissect the language in an ad for skin care products understands what I mean.

As women and as consumers, we don't like to seem gullible. We read the ads, we read the promotional literature, and we shake our heads. It would appear that some of these products are promising to turn back the hands of time. Is that possible? And if it is possible, shouldn't these "scientific breakthroughs" be treated as news items rather than as copy for a skin care line?

Can these new products do everything they claim, or have some of the cosmetics companies gone too far in terms of what they promise? And if the companies are telling the truth and these products can do everything they claim to do, why are they not being called drugs?

Understanding the Difference Between a Drug and a Cosmetic

A cosmetic, as we know, is defined as an article intended to be applied to the human body for cleansing, beautifying, promoting attractiveness, or altering the appearance *without affecting* the body's structure.

A cosmetic *does not* require testing for safety and effectiveness.

On the other hand, products that are intended to treat or prevent disease, or *affect* the structure or functions of the human body, are considered drugs, even when they provide a cosmetic function.

The law in the United States says that products that are intended to *affect* the structure of the human body are required to undergo drug testing for safety and effectiveness even when they provide a cosmetic function.

Cosmetics that are also drugs are usually over-the-counter (OTC) drugs, which can be bought without a prescription. Some examples of over-the-counter drugs that perform a cosmetic function include sunscreens, fluoride toothpaste, hormone creams, and antidandruff shampoos. These products all had to undergo testing for safety and effectiveness.

Why It's Easier to Be Called a Cosmetic

A fact of life that cosmetics companies have long taken for granted, as well as relied upon, is that skin care products and other cosmetics can pretty much be marketed without being cleared by the FDA. Further, so long as they have not been proven harmful they can use almost any ingredients or combination of ingredients without proving that they are effective.

Drugs, on the other hand, are subject to much closer scrutiny. They require premarket approval by the FDA. There are numerous restrictions on the ingredients that can be used. They must be manufactured with certain controls, and, last, but not least, there are rules about the kinds of claims that can be made for drug products—they have to show that they are effective.

Taking into consideration the restrictions that are placed on drugs, even over-the-counter drugs, and the difference in the way the FDA differentiates between cosmetics and drugs, it is easy to see why cosmetics companies are caught in a peculiar bind.

They want consumers to come away with the notion that their skin care products have the power necessary to alter or affect the skin. In other words, if a skin care consumer reads promotional material that makes her believe that a particular product is going to be able to act like a drug and affect the structure of her skin so that it truly has an anti-aging result, this will probably make the consumer buy the product, which is all to their benefit. But, and this is a big but, they don't want to have to live with the kind of testing and regulations that drug status would place on them.

Are Fancy Skin Care Products Drugs or Are They Cosmetics?—The FDA Gets Involved

For many years, the FDA paid little or no attention to the escalating skin care claims. Back in 1984 when I was doing research for my first book, *Save Your Money, Save Your Face,* several people at the FDA told me, off the cuff, that they didn't expect that the FDA would ever get involved in challenging these claims. Essentially, they felt that the FDA had bigger fish to fry, and because of cutbacks and the limitation on its budget, they had to restrict their activities. Safety was quoted as being the major priority. The sense I got was that skin care products, unless they included dangerous ingredients, did not pose immediate health or safety hazards and that the FDA did not have the time or the budget to assume responsibility for protecting the consumer's pocketbook.

Along Came Glycel, Or the Skin Care Claims That Could Not Be Ignored

GSL is perhaps the single most important development in skin care in over a decade.
—PROMOTIONAL MATERIAL FOR GLYCEL GSL CELLULAR LINE

Then came Glycel, a skin care line that many said gave new meaning to the word hype. In early 1986, when Alfin Fragrances launched its Glycel skin care line, the language in the promotional material was so extreme that it forced everyone to begin to look at the claims a little differently. Some of you may remember the original ad with the large bold letters proclaiming "HOW TO GROW YOUNGER SKIN by Dr. Christiaan Barnard." Most of us recognized Dr. Barnard as the South African surgeon who conducted the first successful human heart transplant. The first series of ads said the skin cream "can make older skin behave and look like younger skin." In short, the claims were so extreme that they angered a whole group of people, including fellow cosmetics companies, dermatologists, and some of the trade journals and magazines that cater to the beauty industry.

Several doctors, as well as members of the cosmetics community, openly criticized Dr. Barnard for the way in which he allowed himself to be shown in the Glycel ads. It was their feeling that since he was trained as a surgeon, not as a dermatologist, he was ill-advised to be portrayed as an expert in a field that was not his specialty. Further, many were quick to point out that the ads referred to basic research that had been done for Glycel, but that the manufacturer had done nothing to support its claims by having this research published.

Beauty Fashion, a magazine that caters to the industry, stated their position in an article with the headline ALFIN'S CLAIMS—THE GSL CHARADE, in which it said, "Alfin is the astronaut of skincare claims. They have made a moon landing for pure hype."

It is hard to determine whether it was the extremity of the performance claims or the fact that a well-known medical doctor was associated with them that so annoyed members of the cosmetics community. To people the world over, Christiaan Barnard is respected for his work as a surgical pioneer. But what, more than a few asked, did this have to do with skin care, dermatology, or biochemistry?

The situation was exacerbated by promotional literature that made statements such as "Dr. Barnard has discovered that when aging cells are supplied with GSL, they act young again."

The literature clearly relied upon Dr. Barnard's reputation to create the impression that medical history was again taking place using phrases such as "isolated by Dr. Christiaan Barnard, world-renowned heart surgeon, and a team of Swiss cell biologists." Many of you will remember that the ads also included a diagram of the chemical compound, all very scientific looking, but it made no sense to most skin care consumers.

In interviews at the time, Dr. Barnard, who had retired from surgery because of arthritis, was pictured in a white medical jacket next to a large microscope, thus emphasizing the medical and scientific aspects of the claim.

Further, Glycel claims stated that both GSL and the transdermal carrier used in the products had been granted U.S. patents. Some of Glycel's, and Barnard's, detractors asked, "What patents?" claiming either that they could not find proof of any such patents or that those which had been issued to a biochemist in Switzerland (but not to Dr. Barnard) were not based upon relevant research.

In the beginning, at least, detractors didn't seem to affect Glycel in the slightest. When Glycel launched a nine-product treatment line, they had $5 million in advance sales, and early publicity and Dr. Barnard's involvement had already led to articles in *Newsweek* and *Time*.

The business community had also taken note of Glycel. An article about the product titled "A Skin-Cream Stock That's Working Magic" in the January 13, 1986, issue of *Business Week* featured a photograph of the Glycel packaging and stated, "Early word of a new cosmetic called Glycel sent the stock of Alfin Fragrances Inc. on a ride that carried it to a high of 72 on Dec. 26, nearly three times its price in November. Although the market then cooled off a bit, Alfin was selling in the low 50s on December 30."

Sales in the first few weeks boomed, but some of you may remember that adverse publicity was beginning to emerge. When Glycel's president, Irwin Alfin, an old hand in the cosmetics business (he was former president of Max Factor, Halston, and Chanel Fragrances) appeared on the television show "Nightline," most of us judged the coverage as unfavorable. Initially, however, it seemed to spur sales. And Irwin Alfin hardly seemed disturbed. He even had an answer as to why no scientific publication had taken place and was quoted in *The New York Times* as saying, "We are in a highly competitive business. We're not in the medical field. No one in our industry that we are competing with publishes anything, and therefore we have not and have no plans to."

The exaggeration of the claims, the so-called medical breakthrough, and a sense, as someone said to me, that women would believe anything if it was couched in scientific terms made more than a few people, including several competitors, downright furious.

In July 1986, about six months after Glycel's official launch, when Glycel was talking about reaching up to $10 million in wholesale sales, *Advertising Age* reported that a law firm, acting on behalf of an unidentified client, filed a complaint petitioning the FDA and the FTC to "advise my client . . . how much leeway the commission is prepared to tolerate, so that everyone can play by the same rules." The complaint letter said the Glycel's label claim of rejuvenation rendered the product a "drug within the meaning of the Food, Drug and Cosmetic Act."

Then, another citizen petitioner, assumed to be another skin care manufacturer, asked the FDA to take a stand against yet another anti-aging skin product, this time Avon's BioAdvance. This time it was a little bit different.

With Glycel, part of the complaint indicated that the product was ineffective. With BioAdvance, the complaint stressed the premise that possibly the opposite was true because BioAdvance includes retinol, or Vitamin A, as an ingredient. Retinol is in the same family of ingredients as the anti-acne, antiwrinkle drug marketed by Ortho Pharmaceuticals under the brand name Retin-A. However, retinol and Retin-A are not the same ingredient, and, by now, most of us are aware that Retin-A is available only with a doctor's prescription.

The complaint petition filed with the FDA against BioAdvance asked the FDA to classify the product as a drug. If the FDA acted accordingly, it would, of course, mean that BioAdvance would have to go through all the requirements of new drug testing, a procedure that normally takes as long as ten years, or more.

Enough Is Enough—The FDA Writes a Letter

It wasn't any one claim, or any one product. It was like a mosaic. Take a look at only one stone, and you're not sure of what you see, but when many stones are there, and in place, you can't help but get the picture.

—HEINZ J. EIRMANN,
DIRECTOR, COSMETIC DIVISION, FDA, JUNE, 1987

No one is really sure which product or which set of claims caused the FDA to take action, but in the spring of 1987, the FDA took a long, hard look at the labeling for some of the newer products, and, in essence, they said "enough already," and proceeded to ask the question that skin care consumers had been wondering about for years: If these products can deliver on promotional claims such as cell renewal, anti-aging, antiwrinkling, increased collagen fiber formation, etc., then don't these products really qualify as drugs? And if so, shouldn't they be tested for safety and effectiveness before they are marketed?

In mid-April 1987, the FDA exercised its prerogative and asked the question in earnest. Regulatory letters began to go out to some of the largest firms in the skin care business. The first group of letters was sent to Estée Lauder, Glycel, and Avon. Some people thought that might be it, but within days another group went out, and then another. By the time the FDA was finished, a total of twenty-three skin care manufacturers received regulatory letters.

Among the companies receiving these letters were: Charles of the Ritz for Age-Zone Controller line; Almay for their Skincare for Age-Control Protective Line; The Skin Research Group/Prince Matchabelli for their Dramatic Results Skin Renewal Fluid; Frances Denney for their FD-29 Complete Anti-Aging Complex; Cosmair for their Biotherm line; Jacqueline Cochran for their La Prairie Cellular Skincare line; Pfizer for their Coty Division Overnight Success line; Alfin Fragrances for their Glycel GSL Cellular Products; Estée Lauder for their Night Repair, Eyezone, Skin Perfecting Creme Firming Nourisher, Prescriptives Line Preventor, Estée Lauder Nourishers; Germaine Monteil for their Acti-Vita AntiWrinkle Concentrate; Max Huber Research Labs for their Crème de la Mer; Christian Dior for Capture; Shiseido for B.H.–24 Day/Night Essence; Cosmair for Lancôme's Niosôme; Avon for BioAdvance, Momentum, Night Support, and Collagen Booster; Orlane for Nightly Requirement Creme, Treatment Base Moisture, Morning Recovery Solution, and Hydro Climat; Adrien Arpel for Bio Cellular Plasma Pak + B-12; Clarins for Double Serum Multi-Regenerant Anti-Aging Total Skin Supplement, Fluide Restructurant Restructuring Beauty Treatment, Tenseur Biologique Biological Skin Tightener, and Cellules Fraîches Cell Extracts; Elizabeth Arden for Millennium Day Renewal Emulsion, Millennium Night Renewal Creme, and Visible Difference Refining Moisture Creme Complex; Princess Marcella Borghese for Terme di Montecatini Restorative Fluid for Face and Hydro Minerali Skin Revitalizing Extract; Chanel for Chanel Lift Serum Anti-Wrinkle Complex.

Citing the specific company's specific product claims, the FDA letters stated:

> In summary, the aforementioned claims represent and suggest that the articles are intended to affect the structure and function of the human body, and that the products are adequate and effective for such

uses. . . . Because of such claims, the products are regarded as drugs as defined in section 201(g) of the Federal Food, Drug and Cosmetic Act (Act). Also we are unaware of any substantial scientific evidence that demonstrates the safety and effectiveness of these articles for their intended uses, nor are we aware that these drugs are generally recognized as safe and effective for their intended uses. . . .

The letters reminded the individual companies that it was their responsibility to ensure that all of their products were "the subject of approved new drug applications as appropriate and that the products are properly labeled for their intended uses."

Skin Care Manufacturers in a Quandary

A regulatory letter is a serious matter. It implies that the FDA means business and, if necessary, is prepared to follow up with a regulatory action, which could mean seizure or injunction.

At this point, the skin care companies had to do something, and there were several possibilities open to each manufacturer:

· They could take out all the claims of a physiological nature, leaving only truly cosmetic claims, the advantage being that they wouldn't have to do anything else, and they could just continue to market the product. On the negative side, the consumer has grown accustomed to the promises and the fancy scientific language. What would she think if phrases such as cell renewal, anti-aging, antiwrinkling were replaced by "makes your skin softer and smoother"? Would she be as willing to go out and spend up to $65 an ounce, or more, for a product that promised nothing more complicated than "softer and smoother"?
· They could do nothing, which would mean that the FDA had to act first. The FDA would either have to seize the product or get an injunction to stop the company from distributing the product. The manufacturer could then contest the action and possibly go to court.
· They could stop distributing their product and do what was necessary to get *new drug* status. The problem with this is that once a product is declared a new drug, it can't be marketed until it meets FDA requirements. The process can take ten or twelve years. One can easily see why a manufacturer would prefer not to have its products taken off the counters for this amount of time.

The skin care companies respond: We are not drugs; we are cosmetics, but modern technology has created more effective skin care products, and we want to be able to talk about the technology.

The FDA had not even finished sending out all the regulatory letters when eleven of the first recipients joined together and had their attorneys draft a letter suggesting that all the companies and the FDA work to find a way to "reconcile the benefits of present-day cosmetic science with the Agency's regulatory responsibilities and priorities."

The letter also noted that although there had been tremendous advances in cosmetic science and the development of new products, these advances do not "cause these products to be 'drugs.'"

The FDA responded to this letter by agreeing to meet with the companies that had received regulatory letters. The FDA also requested that the skin care companies submit a "precise written proposal" for review before such a meeting, in the hope that such a proposal would "provide a suitable basis for resolving the matter quickly."

July 20—The First Proposal

Whether the smoothing and plumping are done by traditional moisturizers and smoothing agents, or by the newer products under consideration, the cosmetic benefit is the same: tiny lines temporarily disappear and wrinkles are filled out and appear to diminish, so the user's appearance is improved.

—LETTER TO THE FDA DATED JULY 20, 1987, FROM LEGAL
REPRESENTATIVES OF TWELVE SKIN CARE COMPANIES

The group of skin care companies that decided to act in unison responded by sending off two separate proposals to the FDA, one on July 20 and another, longer one on September 11, 1987.

The first letter asked for flexibility on the part of the FDA and, citing water as an example, stressed the fact that many of the simplest moisturizers affected the structure or function of the body. They pointed out that traditional moisturizers hydrated the surface of the skin, thus plumping up the cells and causing wrinkles to appear less deep—temporarily. According to the July 20 letter, the new products were more sophisticated moisturizers that performed in a more effective manner and did a better job than moisturizers of even the recent past.

However, the letter stressed the fact that this does not mean that these new products are drugs. "In every case, however, no matter how 'high-tech' the product or the words used to describe it, the benefit is cosmetic, just as it was with the moisturizers of old."

The letter also declared that new technology allowed for more advanced methods of measuring the results of skin care products, and promotional material could therefore state with certainty that moisturizers *did* produce an improvement in the appearance of the skin.

Further, although willing to declare certain kinds of claims off-limits, particularly those that products can "reverse or stop the aging process," or those that claim a permanent effect as opposed to an improvement derived from continuous and ongoing use of the products, the skin care companies proposed that they be allowed to continue to include scientific information about skin, and biological processes, such as aging or aging effects of the sun.

July 27—The Meeting

Obviously, I was not present at the July 27, 1987, meeting, but I'm told that the FDA requested that the skin care companies in question make a distinction between physical and physiological effects. In other words, the FDA would find it acceptable if the companies limited themselves and claimed only that their products had a physical effect. They would not allow a product to make claims of a physiological nature. As nearly as I can understand this distinction, by physiological effects the FDA means anything that affects the body below the stratum corneum, or top layer of the epidermis; any effects of a biological nature; or anything that affects a biological function or vital process of the body. By physical, I understand them to mean anything that affects only the surface of the body; anything that involves a mechanical process such as massage or exfoliation of dead skin cells.

September 11—The Second Proposal

As further assurance that cosmetic claims will be limited to the benefits of improved appearance, the undersigned companies will observe two additional general precautions. First, claims or

implications of permanent *benefits (as opposed to continued benefits from repeated use) will not be made. Second, manufacturers will not claim any benefits or effects below the epidermis of the skin.*
—LETTER TO THE FDA DATED SEPTEMBER 11, 1987, FROM LEGAL
REPRESENTATIVES OF ELEVEN MAJOR SKIN CARE COMPANIES

This fifty-four-page-long and thoughtful letter to the FDA from legal representatives of some of the giants in the skin care industry is a fascinating document. It points out that it has been almost twenty years since the FDA last addressed the issue of cosmetics claims. Since then, a great deal has been learned about the way in which skin functions, and this new knowledge makes it difficult if not impossible to separate the stratum corneum from the underlying layers of the epidermis.

Twenty years ago, for example, little was known about the ways in which cosmetic ingredients could penetrate beyond the stratum corneum, and it was believed that the stratum corneum was impenetrable by most substances. Now, of course, we know that many ingredients make it past the stratum corneum into the other layers of the epidermis.

The letter states, among other things, that the stratum corneum and underlying layers of the epidermis interact, and that it is "unrealistic to expect that any cosmetic simply sits on the skin exerting only a physical, transitory effect on the few layers of dead cells atop the stratum corneum."

The letter argues in a fairly sophisticated manner that skin care products should be regarded as cosmetics and not as drugs, because the average consumer realizes that she is purchasing these products simply to enhance her appearance, and that she is not so naive as to believe that these products have a drug effect.

I must admit that I translate this argument to mean that these skin care companies are saying that the consumer doesn't believe their extreme claims, so why should the FDA. This to me seems a trifle odd, but it is less confusing if you understand the reasons for the argument.

In the past, the courts have taken the position that it doesn't matter what the FDA thinks or what the court thinks; what is relevant is how the consumer perceives a product claim.

The skin care companies ended this long letter by offering a compromise that they hoped would be acceptable. Their proposal summarized:

1. The skin care companies won't claim that their products affect the aging process by slowing it down or reversing it. However, they could use anti-aging and prevention claims in promoting sunscreens, as in "to help prevent premature aging of the skin."

2. Skin care companies could truthfully discuss the aging process and inform consumers of biological processes so long as these statements are truthful and not misleading and did not connect these processes with the use of their products.
3. The skin care companies could truthfully claim that their products improved the appearance of the skin and made it look younger so long as they did not imply that these effects were permanent or that they affected the skin below the epidermis.

The FDA Responds

When the FDA responded to the proposal submitted by the attorneys for the skin care companies, it became apparent that no amount of complicated language was going to convince them that skin care products could point to physiological results and still maintain cosmetic status.

> We consider a claim that a product will affect the body in some physiological way to be a drug claim, even if the claim is only temporary. . . . For example, claims that a product "counteracts," "retards," or "controls" aging or the aging process, as well as claims that a product will "rejuvenate," "repair," or "renew" the skin are drug claims because they can be fairly understood as claims that a function of the body, or that the structure of the body, will be affected by the product. For this reason also, all of the examples that you use to allege an effect within the epidermis as the basis for a temporary beneficial effect on wrinkles, lines, or fine lines are unacceptable. A claim such as "molecules absorb . . . and expand, exerting upward pressure to 'lift' wrinkles upward" is a claim for an inner, structural change.

Representatives of the FDA have made it clear that they believe that most, if not all, of these products provide only a cosmetic function, as is evident in their letter, which says, "While we agree with your statements that wrinkles will not be reversed or removed by these products . . ." However, the FDA is also making it clear that they consider many of the *claims* that skin care manufacturers are making cause the products to fall into the drug category; the letter goes on to say, "Products that actually affect the structure and any function of the body in the many ways you describe surely require a close and careful scrutiny by FDA to assure their safety."

By the end of this letter, there is no confusion over the seriousness of the FDA's intent. The closing paragraph states: "We believe that FDA has extended an adequate opportunity for a response to our regulatory letters. Accordingly, unless each firm responds individually within 30 days as to the measures that it will take to correct the violations cited in the regulatory letter that it received, the agency will take such action as it deems necessary to resolve its regulatory concerns."

What It All Means for the Skin Care Consumer

The consumer is already beginning to see changes in the advertisements for skin care products. Although it is doubtful that skin care companies are going to let go of their "scientific" skin care pitch, the FDA's position is going to force most of them to tone down some of the more exaggerated promotional and labeling language. Unless the product contains a valid anti-aging ingredient such as a sunscreen, companies are going to be very careful about making anti-aging claims. However, companies can legitimately add sunscreen ingredients that have proven to be safe and effective to a traditional moisturizer and make an anti-aging claim.

Because the FDA is carefully watching the printed word, what we may see happening now is that more companies will feature semiscientific skin care "clinics" within department stores as major promotions. Instead of being blitzed by the ads, you now will be blitzed inside the store with computers, minispas, cameras, etc.

Some companies are continuing to circulate skin information as well as customer follow-up information. The cosmetic salesperson is often trained in a certain amount of scientific jargon, much of which often gets totally confused when it is being repeated to the skin care consumer.

Skin care companies are not ready to give up on the scientific approach. Some companies say they will not let the matter rest. Estée Lauder, for example, has indicated that it is prepared to pursue it further, stating that modern technology has advanced and that the FDA should alter its attitude to allow for an explanation of that technology in the company's literature. Nonetheless, most companies are beginning to modify their labeling to avoid serious confrontation with the FDA. In the meantime, Glycel, the company that started most of this, failed to overwhelm the skin care consumer and, after the FDA action, appears to have stopped distributing its products.

Temporary—A Word for Consumers to Keep in Mind

In this exchange of letters between the FDA and representatives of large skin care lines, the consumer can see how far the skin care companies are prepared to go to defend their anti-aging claims, and how they realistically evaluate the effects that their products have.

The ads have confused many women who wondered whether the visible results to be derived from one of these contemporary skin care products were durable, or like lipstick or foundation makeup, was it just a cosmetic, and temporary, improvement.

The most interesting thing to me about this initial response from the skin care companies was that to date they acknowledged that the results, or benefits, to be obtained from even the most advanced products available today would be temporary in nature.

However, I think it is equally important for the skin care consumer to realize that, all things being equal, the woman who practices long-term preventive skin care, including the regular use of sunscreen products, is more likely to end up at fifty, sixty, seventy, or even eighty with better-looking skin.

10

Talking About Sunscreens

How I Found Happiness While Protecting My Skin Against UVB

My husband is a very practical businessman who is not given to flights of fantasy or illogical thoughts. However, many years ago he was with friends at a state fair, and they happened upon the traditional gypsy fortune teller. Because she claimed to have great psychic abilities, and they had an hour to kill before they could leave, my future husband and his friends had their fortunes told. Here's what she said to him: "I see the woman you will marry. She is facing away from you, but she is turning toward you—slowly, slowly. As she turns, I see her nose outlined in white." Norman and his friends laughed a lot, and he forgot about it until. . . . years later when I was standing on a beach in Florida. I was wearing a nifty little yellow two-piece bathing suit, and because the day before I had spent too much time in the sun, I was worried about burning. This was before sunblocks and sunscreens had become popular. So to protect myself, I had completely covered my nose with zinc oxide, which, as most of you know, looks like a thick, shiny white paste. Suddenly I heard footsteps behind me, and I turned. Guess who it was?

Well, reader, we were married a year later. My husband says that despite the yellow bathing suit, he might not have stopped if it hadn't been for the fact that my nose was outlined with a white sunscreen.

I wish I could promise all of you that all you have to do to find happiness and love is wear a sunscreen. I can't. However, I can promise you that avoiding the sun's ultraviolet rays will protect your skin in the following two ways:

1. Prevent the premature wrinkling and aging that is caused by sun damage.

Some dermatologists feel that sun damage is responsible for as much as 90 percent of all wrinkling, and all experts agree that ultraviolet rays from the sun are the primary culprits involved in causing premature aging of the skin; protecting your skin from these rays can help you avoid sagging skin, wrinkling skin, and collagen breakdown.

2. Help you prevent the most common forms of skin cancer.

If you spent little time in the sun, both as a child and an adult, your chances of developing basal skin cancer are about one in a hundred. However, if your parents took you to the beach as a toddler, and you developed a fondness for sun-related activities that stayed with you as an adult, your chances of developing skin cancer go up to as much as one in four. Protecting your skin from solar rays will significantly reduce the risk of developing skin cancer.

I must admit that I was not too bright about the sun when I was younger. My generation did not receive adequate warnings about the dangers of too much sun, and like many of my peers, I spent an excessive amount of time sunbathing. Consequently, some of my skin, particularly on my arms and legs, has sun damage.

I've had several friends who have had skin cancer, and all of them have been sun worshippers who discovered the facts too late. When I think of the way my generation used to mix iodine with baby oil and then sit out to fry, I shudder. My daughters and their friends are better informed. However, many of them are still confused about the possibility of sun damage and are prepared to forego wisdom in favor of bronzed skin. I certainly can sympathize with the sentiments involved in wanting a beautiful tan. However, I am convinced that paler is better and that staying that way will ultimately pay off in smoother, younger-looking skin.

Fortunately there are now many products available that can be used to shield your skin from the sun. Unfortunately, trying to decide what to use is often confusing and time-consuming. Here are some facts to help you protect your skin from the photoaging effects of the sun.

Sunburn

The technical term for sunburn is erythema. All that means is that the skin is inflamed and presents a flushed, red appearance. This painful reaction is the result of sun damage. Excessive exposure to the sun's ultraviolet light causes many different reactions in the skin. In the epidermis, cells are killed off prematurely, and damaged cells cluster together to form "sunburn" cells.

A change in the pigmentation of our skin is what we notice first. The epidermis starts to thicken, and the skin begins to lay down melanin at a faster pace. Immediate pigment darkening is the result of an alteration in the melanin that is already present in our skin. Delayed tanning is the result of increased epidermal melanin. If you are fair, sometimes the melanin goes down in an uneven fashion, and a blotchy type of pigmentation, otherwise known as freckles, is formed. In the dermis, the volume of blood present increases, causing swelling and edema.

The severity of the sunburn depends upon how sun-sensitive the skin is and how long it has been exposed. Many of us are only too familiar with the pain, blistering, and subsequent peeling that accompany a severe sunburn.

If you are exposed for only a short time, and you are fortunate, your only symptom might be a light, flushed appearance that disappears within a couple of days. In more severe cases, after exposure, the skin may appear almost bright red, and pain, tenderness, and swelling are present.

Symptoms of a sunburn usually appear within one to twenty-four hours, and, unless it is a very bad burn, can be expected to pass the peak of pain and discomfort within two or three days. What often happens then is that the damaged skin begins to scale off or peel. The fairer the skin, the more severe the burn, and the longer it can last. Some very fair-skinned individuals have reported symptoms of sunburn that have lasted for weeks.

If the burn is not severe, the sunburn will fade over several days, leaving behind a skin that is tanned.

Sun Damage Is Cumulative

By the time most of us hit our thirties, we will have spent enough time in the sun to destroy skin cells as well as damage collagen and elastin fibers.

The process by which skin is damaged by the sun is known as photoaging. The changes in the skin that occur as a result of photoaging are not exactly the same as those that occur during the normal aging process, and some prominent dermatologists believe that photoaging is responsible for most wrinkling as well as other types of skin damage such as yellowing, drying, discoloring, thickening, hardening, etc.

In photoaging, for example, the elastic fibers deteriorate at a much faster rate, with more extreme results and a greater loss of elasticity. In normal aging, collagen becomes more stable; in photoaging, collagen decreases. In normal aging, the epidermis becomes thinner; in photoaging, the epidermis thickens, causing a more leathery look. And, in photoaging, blood vessels and Langerhans cells are damaged at a much faster rate.

Every time you sit in the sun, you damage your skin. How much damage depends on how strong the sun's rays are and how long you stay in the sun. It may take ten years or more before photoaging changes are visible to the naked eye.

And even more disturbing than the photoaging effects of the sun are the statistics concerning skin cancer in this country. About half a million new cases are reported each year, and the sun is implicated in at least 90 percent of them.

There are five realistic concerns about the damaging effects of the sun:

1. Acute sunburn reaction.
2. Photoaging from repeated exposure to ultraviolet rays.
3. Precancerous and cancerous malignancies of the skin.
4. Damage to the eyes caused by solar radiation.
5. Alteration of the immune system caused by damage to Langerhans cells in the skin and possible immune incompetence.

The best way to protect your skin from the sun is to stay out of it. Some dermatologists feel so strongly about this that they recommend that their patients never, ever sit in the sun, even with a sunscreen. One I spoke to went so far as to suggest that her patients never even walk on the sunny side of the street.

There are, of course, people who absolutely cannot imagine avoiding direct sunlight. They include those who work outdoors and are constantly exposed to the sun, those who are devoted to outdoor athletic activities, and those to whom nothing is more appealing than long summer afternoons at the local beach.

For those folks (and I'm one of them), God gave us sunscreens. Sunscreens, properly applied, provide reasonably effective protection against the harmful effects of solar radiation.

A Sunscreen Is a Drug, Not a Cosmetic

A sunscreen is a product that is designed to help mitigate the damage caused by the effects of ultraviolet radiation from the sun's rays on skin. These products contain ingredients that are classified as sunscreen agents and that work by either reflecting, absorbing, or scattering ultraviolet light.

Since 1978 the FDA has classified products containing sunscreen agents as over-the-counter drugs and not as cosmetics. This means the active ingredients in sunscreen products must undergo testing for safety and effectiveness for their intended use before they can be marketed. Only FDA-approved sunscreen ingredients can make claims concerning protection from sunburn, premature aging, and skin cancer. Consumers can shop for sunscreens knowing that some degree of caution has been taken for their protection.

How Sunscreens Work

Sunscreens work by protecting your skin from solar energy. When reading sunscreen advertisements, you see the initials UVB and sometimes UVA. The UV is an abbreviation for *u*ltrav*i*olet, meaning the ultraviolet rays that are emitted by the sun. These rays are classified by wavelength as A, B, or C.

UVC, the short-wavelength rays, do not reach the earth; most of them are absorbed by the ozone layer in the earth's upper atmosphere. Therefore, sunscreen products don't take UVC into consideration.

UVA represents the long-wavelength rays, once considered as the "safe" tanning rays. New information suggests that too much UVA exposure may be as damaging as UVB exposure. Although UVA rays do not produce as serious a sunburn as UVB, they penetrate more deeply into the dermis and exposure to them can lead to long-range skin damage.

UVB rays, the "tanning" rays, are responsible for most sunburns. These rays reach us all year round and deliver ultraviolet to the stratum corneum as well as the superficial layers of the epidermis.

There are two types of sunscreens:

1. Physical sunscreens.
   A sunscreen may work by forming an actual physical barrier against the rays of the sun. These products, known as physical sunscreens, do not

absorb ultraviolet rays; instead, they work by scattering and reflecting them. Only two chemicals are approved as physical sunscreen ingredients: red petrolatum and titanium dioxide.

2. Chemical sunscreens.

A chemical sunscreen works by absorbing some, but not all, of the ultraviolet rays. The majority of the sunscreens that we use are chemical sunscreens.

The majority of the approved chemical sunscreens can be broken down into four main categories of active ingredients: PABA and PABA esters (including glyceryl PABA, padimate A, and octyl dimethyl PABA, also known as padimate O), benzophenones, cinnamates, and anthranilates.

PABA, the PABA esters, and the cinnamates protect only against UVB. The benzophenones (oxybenzone, methoxybenzone, and sulfisobenzone) primarily protect against UVA. The anthranilates are moderately effective protection against both UVA and UVB.

Understanding SPF

SPF stands for sun protection factor. This index defines the amount of solar energy required to produce a minimal sunburn on sunscreen-protected skin compared to the amount of solar energy required to produce the same level of sunburn on unprotected skin. The higher the SPF number, the more protection it should afford from exposure to UVB rays. The FDA designates five degrees of protection according to the product's sun protection factor (SPF):

Degree of Protection	SPF
Minimal sun protection	2–4
Moderate sun protection	4–6
Extra sun protection	6–8
Maximal sun protection	8–15
Ultra sun protection	15 or greater

The number gives you some sense of how long you can stay in the sun without becoming sunburned. If you burn easily and would normally start to turn red after ten minutes in the sun and you purchased a number 15 sunscreen, you should be able to stay in the sun 150 minutes, or two and a half hours, before you get the same level sunburn:

Burn Time Without Sunscreen		*SPF*		*Burn Time With Sunscreen*
10 minutes	$\times$	15	$=$	150 minutes (2½ hrs.)

What SPF Is Right for You

How badly or how gracefully you tan or burn is largely a matter of genetics and skin color. Experts classify our individual sensitivity to the sun by our suntanning history and the color of our unexposed body skin. To figure out the color of your unexposed body skin, they take a look at the shade of skin on your buttocks. Using this color and suntanning history, they have come up with the following six sun skin types:

Type 1 has white unexposed skin, is very sensitive to the sun, always burns easily, and never tans.

Type 2 has white unexposed skin, is very sensitive to the sun, always burns easily, and tans minimally.

Type 3 has white unexposed skin, is sensitive to the sun, burns moderately, and tans gradually and uniformly.

Type 4 has light-brown unexposed skin, is moderately sensitive to the sun, burns minimally, and always tans well.

Type 5 has brown unexposed skin, is minimally sensitive to the sun, rarely burns, and tans profusely.

Type 6 has dark-brown or black unexposed skin, is insensitive to the sun, has skin that is deeply pigmented, and never burns.

Before you begin picking and choosing your SPF numbers, I think I should tell you that the Skin Cancer Foundation, as well as many dermatologists, suggests that just about everyone use a sunscreen with an SPF of 15. There are a number of sunscreens with SPFs of 15 and higher that bear the Skin Cancer Foundation Seal of Acceptance. These are the products that have met the sunscreen criteria of the Foundation's Photobiology Committee.

Cosmetics manufacturers often use the following criteria to determine how easily a person burns and what strength SPF should be used:

Skin Type	Degree of Sensitivity	SPF
1 and 2	Very sensitive	15 or higher
3	Sensitive	10–15
4	Moderately sensitive	6–10
5	Minimally sensitive	4–6
6	Not sensitive	None

If you have darker skin, you are obviously less likely to burn, but overexposure to ultraviolet rays can still cause damage, including premature aging and skin cancer. Several dermatologists have advised me that the newest information linking ultraviolet A with long-term skin damage is such that all women, including those with very dark-brown or black skin, should be wearing a protective sunscreen.

You Can Burn Even Though You Are Wearing a Sunscreen   Assuming that a sunscreen provides total protection is a common mistake. Assuming that a sunscreen means that you will only tan, not burn, is another common mistake. Not so. You can still burn; it just takes longer.

The SPF is not calculated for the length of time it takes you to *tan*. It is calculated for the time it takes you to *burn*, so don't think that if you have sensitive skin you can apply a 10 sunscreen and hang out in the sun for a couple of hours without getting a sunburn.

When the SPF Is Above 15   Some companies now manufacture sunscreens with SPFs that reach as high as 29. There is some conflict about the validity of these higher SPFs.

Some experts point out that the only people for whom these higher SPFs have any real value are those who are extraordinarily sun-sensitive, and they probably shouldn't be in the sun under any circumstances. They say that for the normally sun-sensitive person, an SPF of 15 should be more than efficient, and anything more than that is just playing an unnecessary numbers game.

Other experts disagree, maintaining that the higher numbers provide better protection. Dr. Albert Kligman, the highly respected dermatologist who did the initial research on Retin-A and aging, told me that he thought that the higher SPFs were advisable, particularly for fair-skinned women who indulged in outdoor sports such as tennis, swimming, and skiing.

Water-Resistant/Waterproof Because sunscreens are over-the-counter drugs, there are certain standards that must be maintained in claims. I'm always confused by the difference between water-resistant and water-proof, but the FDA is very precise in what standards a product has to meet before these claims can be made. What precisely does "waterproof" mean and how resistant is "water-resistant"?

Manufacturers test their product this way: Sunscreen is applied to a subject, who undergoes a series of twenty-minute water immersions. The subject engages in moderate activity during each immersion, such as swimming or walking through a pool.

The number of twenty-minute immersions without the sunscreen washing off defines the possible claim. "Water-resistant" means two immersions, for a total of forty minutes. "Waterproof" means four immersions and eighty minutes in the water.

Shopping for Sunscreens

Purchasing the right sunscreen requires thought and careful consideration. If your local store doesn't have the product you want in the formula that is right for your skin, take the time to shop around and get the product you want. It will be worth it. If you find the product you like at the beginning of the summer, buy several bottles. Stores often run out and don't always replace stock until the next season.

A problem I have found in shopping for sunscreens is limited selection of SPF and brand names. Many times the products that are available aren't brand new. This is important because many companies have recently changed their formulas to protect against both UVB and UVA.

Also, some companies offer noncomedegenic or extramoisturizing formulas that offer a choice beyond just SPF.

Here's a list of qualities to take into consideration when you shop for sunscreens:

1. SPF number.

I always buy several sunscreens with different SPFs for different purposes.

2. Type of UV screen.

With the new information that links UVA to skin cancer as well as to long-term damage of dermal tissue, I think it's best to make certain that the sunscreen protects against both UVB and UVA. If it does, it will almost certainly list this protection on the label.

3. Alcohol or nonalcohol base.

Yes, skin type is important even with sunscreens. Many offer noncomedegenic formulas, which is great for the woman with oily or acne-prone skin. What few women realize, however, is that there are sunscreens with different formulas for different skin types.

Sunscreens that have an alcohol base are often better suited for oily skin. Other sunscreens are creams and are better suited for dry skin.

Most of the time you can tell the difference by looking at the sunscreen. The alcohol-based ones are often clear, while the creams look like creams. The trick is trying to figure out whether the product is right for you before you buy it. Here are some clues: Alcohol-based sunscreens will often use words like "cool alcohol formula." Nonalcohol-based sunscreens will often use the words "oil" or "cream." Sometimes you have to read all the small print on the back of the package to find these words. Alcohol-based sunscreens are also less likely to be waterproof than are nonalcoholic ones.

Some companies manufacture products with the same SPFs, but in different formulas. An example is Westwood's PreSun, which can be found in Creamy (waterproof), Lotion (for normal to oily skin), and Facial (designed not to cause acne or blemishes) formulas.

4. Waterproof or nonwaterproof.

If you are a swimmer, you are a lot safer using waterproof sunscreen—for the obvious reasons. Also you should know that the sun's rays reach into the water itself, so the fact that you are underwater is no protection. But remember that waterproof sunscreens are more apt to be cream or oil-based, and this may be a consideration if you have oily skin.

Getting a Sunscreen in Moisturizers and Other Cosmetics

Choose a sunscreen to get the best protection available. Manufacturers include sunscreens in some moisturizer and foundation products. This allows the companies to make claims such as "protects from premature aging." When these products do include sunscreens, concentrations may be too low to provide adequate protection. If a product has an approved sunscreen ingredient, it should be classified as an over-the-counter drug and the SPF should also be listed. If it is a cosmetic and not an over-the-counter drug, it has not received approval for safety and efficacy. If a product has a high enough SPF to protect your skin from the sun, and you want to use it to increase your sun protection, remember to reapply it at regular intervals.

Foundations That Include Sunscreens There are some foundation makeups that include chemical physical sunscreens. Two opaque make-ups are: Clinique's Continuous Coverage and Lydia O'Leary's Cover-Mark. If your facial skin is very sensitive to sunscreen ingredients with high SPFs, these can be used, preferably with a sunscreen lotion (with as strong an SPF as you can manage). Remember with these foundations that application is the key to protection. Cover your entire face and neck with a smooth, even cover of the foundation. When using these foundations for sun protection, apply carefully, making sure that you haven't missed any exposed areas including the tips and tops of the ears, under the eyes, etc. Reapply the foundation at regular intervals, and don't forget that they are not waterproof and that perspiration and water will remove them.

Some Sunscreens and Some Ingredients Here are the ingredients currently listed in some popular sunscreens. I'm including these only so that you can become accustomed to looking at sunscreen ingredients before you buy the product. Notice that the lotions, rather than the creams, are more likely to include alcohol. Also notice that there are different formulas manufactured by the same company so that you can't make generalities about which ones are best for you without reading the ingredients. If your pharmacy doesn't stock products that are PABA-free or designed for sensitive skin, have them order one for you. Formulas often change, so you have to check the ingredients label every time you make a purchase.

Sundown Sunscreen Ultra Protection (SPF 24, cream)—padimate O and oxybenzone

Sundown Ultra Protection (SPF 20, lotion)—padimate O, octyl methoxycinnamate, oxybenzone, titanium dioxide, and benzyl alcohol

Block Out by Sea & Ski (SPF 15, cream)—padimate O, octyl methoxycinnamate, and oxybenzone

Block Out Clear by Sea & Ski (SPF 15, lotion)—padimate O, octyl methoxycinnamate, octyl salicylate, and SD alcohol 40

PreSun 15 Creamy (SPF 15, cream)—padimate O and oxybenzone

PreSun 15 (SPF 15, lotion)—padimate O, oxybenzone, PABA and SD alcohol 40

Solbar Plus 15 (SPF 15, cream)—padimate O, oxybenzone, and dioxybenzone

Solbar (SPF 15, cream)—octyl methoxycinnamate and oxybenzone (PABA-free)

Water Babies Sunblock by Coppertone (SPF 15, lotion)—ethylhexyl-P-methoxycinnamate and oxybenzone

Physical Sunscreens If you want to be extra sure that your skin is protected, you might want to consider using a physical sunscreen such as zinc oxide or a product containing titanium dioxide for extrasensitive areas.

How to Apply Sunscreen

My friend Sally has fair skin and brunette hair. Recently she planned a trip to the beach, and she wisely made a drugstore visit and selected a water-resistant sunscreen with an SPF of 15. As soon as she hit the sand, she covered herself with the sunscreen. When she got home late that afternoon, she discovered that she had a very mild sunburn. This was nothing disastrous, but it was more than she expected. She called me that evening to ask me how the sun could have penetrated a sunscreen with an SPF of 15.

Sally made at least one major mistake in applying her sunscreen. She waited until she was on the beach before using it. It takes at least fifteen to thirty minutes for the chemicals in many sunscreens to penetrate the top layer of skin, and in Sally's case, she was unprotected for more minutes than her fair skin could afford.

Here are some suggestions for applying sunscreen.

1. *Don't* apply sunscreen to skin that is inflamed or eczematous without consulting a physician.
2. Apply the sunscreen at least thirty minutes before you go out into the sun.
3. Be certain that you are applying enough of it. When companies test sunscreen products for the degree of protection or SPF that they give, the sunscreen product is applied very liberally. You can't skimp on sunscreen.
4. Reapply sunscreen at regular intervals, and don't run the risk of perspiration leaving your skin unprotected.
5. If you are not using a waterproof product, reapply the product whenever you go into the water.

More facts about sunburns:

· You can burn at any time of the day, but the sun is strongest between 10 A.M. and 3 P.M.
· You can get a burn even on the haziest days because ultraviolet rays easily pass through the haze.
· If you are at a high altitude, you have a greater chance of burning; there is less atmosphere to absorb the sun's rays.
· The closer you are to the equator, the more likely you are to burn.
· Sitting under an umbrella at the beach does not guarantee protection; both sand and water reflect the sun's rays, so that a shady spot does not mean you don't need a sunscreen.
· The sun's rays not only reflect off water, but also can pass through it—up to three feet; keep that in mind when you are swimming.

Do Black Women Need a Sunscreen? I've spoken to several dermatologists about the effects of ultraviolet light on black skin, and they basically feel that black women should not risk the possibility of damage from ultraviolet A by not using a sunscreen. Also, black skin needs protection because it is prone to exaggerated pigment responses, some of which are directly related to sun exposure. You don't need as much protection as a woman with fair skin, and, depending upon your skin tone, you can stick to the lower SPFs. When choosing your sunscreen, always remember to take your skin type into consideration.

Does a Tan Protect Your Skin from Sunburn? Yes, but it doesn't protect it from sun damage or skin cancer. Remember that a tan is the skin's protective reaction to injury from ultraviolet light. Believing that an already-acquired tan will protect your skin from photoaging is false.

Nonsunscreen Suntan Lotions and Oils Not all suntan lotions and oils are sunscreens. Some, in fact, are designed to increase the amount of tan you get. Just because a product says it is suntan lotion or suntan oil does not mean it is a sunscreen. A sunscreen product will always refer to itself as a sunscreen, not a lotion, and it will carry an SPF number.

Trying Out Your Sunscreen Before You Go to the Beach

So many women have told me variations on this story that I think it is important to repeat this story, which was told to me by a close friend.

> Last June my husband and I decided to take a trip to an out-of-the-way beach in Montauk. It was a beautiful day, and we drove the two or so hours. On the way, I stopped at a drugstore to buy some sunscreen. They didn't have the brand that I had been using for years, but I bought another one with an SPF of 15. We got to the beach, and I put on the screen. Within minutes, my skin felt as though it was on fire. I was fortunate that the beach had a water fountain, and I washed off my face, but no matter how much water I used, my skin still felt totally irritated. And then, of course, I was concerned that I was not protected and would get a sunburn. We had to leave the beach, drive to the nearest town, and find another product. I put it on my face, which was still uncomfortable. All in all, the experience turned what should have been a lovely day at the beach into a series of small disasters.

I always advise women to buy the sunscreen they plan to use weeks before they will need to use it and apply it at various times and leave it on to make certain that the product doesn't irritate the skin.

Some women complain about sensitivity to sunscreen ingredients. If you are one of them, the search to find a product that does not irritate your skin is one of trial and error. If your skin becomes irritated from a sunscreen, the first thing to do is to write down the list of ingredients. Take a look at the sunscreen ingredient itself. PABA and PABA esters, particularly glyceryl PABA, are often accused of being weak allergens, but remember that even if you are allergic or sensitive to one form of PABA, that does not mean you will respond the same way to all of them. Some women react to other sunscreens. Take a look, also, at the other ingredients. Your reaction may be caused by one of them. Fragrances or preservatives are always a possibility. Another thing to consider is that it may be something totally different irritating your skin. You may have dry skin and have purchased a sunscreen with an alcohol base that is drying and irritating your skin.

The next time you go shopping for a sunscreen, take your list of ingredients in the offending product with you. This time, when you buy a product, choose one with a different sunscreen ingredient. Some companies do advertise that their products are less likely to cause a reaction, and when searching for a sunscreen product, you should probably start with some of these products.

Stronger SPFs Cause a Burning or Itching Sensation

> I have been using the SPF number 8 in a particular sunscreen line for years, and I really like the products. However, whenever I try to use one of their products with an SPF number 15, my face starts to burn and itch. What do I do?

The higher the SPF, the greater the concentration of active ingredients, and this may be causing the irritation. When this happens, try an SPF number 15 in a brand that has different active ingredients.

Of course, the possibility exists that it may be an entirely different ingredient that has been added to the higher SPF, so read the label carefully.

If you absolutely cannot find a product with a high SPF that doesn't irritate your skin, then start experimenting with lower SPFs. You may find that you are less sensitive to the lower concentrations.

However, you must remember that you will not be as well protected, and you should compensate for that with clothing and hats. You may want to try a combination of a lower SPF sunscreen *plus* a foundation makeup that contains a physical opaque sunscreen such as titanium dioxide on your face and other sun-sensitive parts of your body. (See the list at the end of this chapter.) If you are forced to use a lower SPF, don't go into the sun during the midday hours, and do compensate with clothing and umbrellas. It's also extra important with the lower SPFs to reapply the sunscreen at regular intervals.

Women who have this type of sensitivity usually find that it is limited only to the facial area. They can, *and should*, continue to use high SPFs on their bodies.

Photoallergies and Photosensitivity

A photoallergy or photosensitivity occurs when certain chemicals, either applied to the body or ingested as drugs or other substances, interact with rays from the sun. Unfortunately some of the substances are themselves sunscreen ingredients, such as PABA esters, Para-aminobenzoic acid, benzophenones, cinnamates, and oxybenzone. Drugs that may cause photosensitive reactions include:

antibiotics, such as the tetracylines

anticancer drugs, such as dacarbazine

antidepressants

antihistamines

antimicrobials, such as demeclocycline (Declomycin and others) and nalidixic acid (NegGram)

antiparasitic drugs, such as bithionol (Bitin)

antipsychotic drugs

diuretics, such as Diuril, HydroDIURIL, and Lasix

fragrances and perfumes

halogenated salicylanilides, including ones found in antiseptics and some deodorant soaps

hypoglycemics

nonsteroid anti-inflammatory drugs, such as piroxicam

sulfonamides, such as sulfadiazine, sulfathiazole, sulfanilamide, and others

Some photosensitivity reactions are mild, but sometimes they can be more severe. The most common involve a sunburn-like reaction with redness, swelling, blisters, peeling, etc. However, there is a photoallergic reaction that looks like a contact dermatological reaction with rashes or wheels.

Don't use local anesthetics with a photosensitive reaction and call your doctor to get his advice on how to treat it. He may suggest something as simple as cool baths and compresses or he may feel that you require a prescription drug and an office visit.

Tanning Salons and Home Tanning Equipment

They get a negative vote. When these salons first opened up, most of them used equipment that emitted only ultraviolet B. Then it became increasingly apparent that UVB was connected to skin damage and skin cancer. So many of them switched equipment, concentrated on UVA, and outfitted themselves with lamps that emitted mostly ultraviolet A. Because ultraviolet A can give a tan without burning, it seemed so appealing, and easy. Unfortunately, it was no solution. Ultraviolet A poses more than a few problems. It penetrates more deeply into the skin than UVB and ultimately can age your skin and add wrinkles just as effectively as UVB.

Because of the high intensity of the UVA equipment, there is, of course, special concern for people who don't tan and always burn (type 1 and type 2). There is also some concern about adverse cutaneous drug photosensitivity reactions in anyone receiving therapeutic medication for a range of medical problems, including hypertension, bacterial infections, diabetes, and cardiac, renal, and mental disorders. Obviously, patients with diseases that are exacerbated by sunlight such as lupus or an already existing history of skin cancer are at particular risk from exposure to UVA equipment.

As for skin cancer and UVA, all the evidence is not in. There are some experts who feel that UVA is not directly implicated in basal cell carcinoma of the skin. However, they feel that there is some evidence that heavily implicates UVA rays in melanoma, which is the more serious form of skin cancer.

It has been shown that UVA can cause serious and painful problems for the eyes. Long-term exposure, for example, may cause cataracts and chronic corneal problems.

Protecting the eyes is something that people who buy sunlamps for home use often forget about. Closing the eyes is no protection against the ultraviolet rays. There is a reason why tanning salons use goggles, and they are absolutely necessary.

The Food and Drug Administration is so convinced of the hazards of using ultraviolet radiation to get a tan that regulations were recently amended and now suntanning equipment such as beds and booths must carry the following warning statements:

> DANGER. Ultraviolet Radiation. Follow instructions. Avoid overexposure. As with natural sunlight, overexposure can cause eye and skin injury and allergic reactions. Repeated exposure may cause premature aging of the skin and skin cancer. Wear protective eyewear: Failure to do so may result in severe burns or long-term injury to the eyes. Medications or cosmetics may increase your sensitivity to ultraviolet radiation. Consult your physician before using a sunlamp if you are using medications or have a history of skin problems or believe yourself to be especially sensitive to the sunlight. If you do not tan in the sun, you are unlikely to tan from the use of this product.

Skin Cancer

No discussion of the sun's effects on the skin can go without a warning about skin cancer. Here are some facts to consider:

Basal Skin Cancer

This is the most common form of skin cancer, and each year it affects approximately 400,000 Americans. Most of you will remember that former president Ronald Reagan developed basal skin cancer on the tip of his nose. As a matter of fact, one in eight Americans will develop this type of skin cancer, and most cases are attributed to overexposure to sunlight. It is believed that people with fair skin, light hair, and blue, green, or gray eyes are at highest risk.

Basal skin cancer is most likely to occur on exposed parts of the body such as the face, ears, neck, scalp, shoulders, and back (there are, however, some rare instances in which it develops on nonexposed areas).

Anyone can get basal cell carcinoma, but the most likely candidates are those who are regularly exposed to the sun. This includes workers in occupations that require long hours outdoors as well as sports and sun enthusiasts whose leisure hours bring them into heavy contact with the sun's rays.

As you might expect, the incidence of basal cell carcinoma increases as you get closer to the equator. Basal cell carcinoma can be quite deceptive and may mimic a noncancerous skin condition such as psoriasis or eczema. A trained dermatologist is best qualified to make the distinction. The warning signs are:

· *an open sore* that bleeds, oozes, or crusts and remains open for three or more weeks. A persistent, nonhealing sore is a very common sign of an early basal cell carcinoma.
· *a reddish patch* or irritated area, frequently occurring on the chest, shoulders, arms, or legs. Sometimes the patch crusts. It may also itch or hurt. At other times, it persists with no noticeable discomfort.
· *a smooth growth* with an elevated, rolled border, and an indentation in the center. As the growth slowly enlarges, tiny blood vessels may develop on the surface.
· *a shiny bump,* or nodule, that is pearly or translucent and is often pink, red, or white. The bump can also be tan, black, or brown, especially in dark-haired people, and can be confused with a mole.
· *a scar-like area*—white, yellow, or waxy—which often has poorly defined borders. The skin itself appears shiny and taut. Although a less frequent sign of a cancer, it can indicate the presence of an aggressive tumor.

Both basal cell carcinoma and squamous cell carcinoma are very easily treated when the carcinoma is detected and removed in its early stages. Untreated, however, it can necessitate extensive and potentially disfiguring surgery, although it will rarely become life threatening.

Basal Cell Carcinoma—One Woman's Story

The following story was told to me by a New York writer, who wrote about her experiences in greater depth for various publications. She wants to share her experience because she is so acutely aware of how easy it is to let skin cancer go unnoticed and untreated.

I always thought of myself as a darkish-skinned person, and I never burned—I always tanned. I didn't know then what I know now: that although a tan keeps you from burning, it doesn't protect you from skin cancer.

I always loved the water. As a child I spent time at lakes and ponds, and then later I spent time in Europe and vacationed on the Mediterranean. One year, when I was in my thirties, I noticed that my nose was red. Not flaming red, just a little pinkish. I showed it to several doctors, but I didn't go to a dermatologist. Basically, I walked around with a red nose for about three years. During that time I visited several doctors for other reasons, and I would always ask them about my nose. One of them even said that it was just veins. Then one summer it started to bleed and, finally, I went to a dermatologist who told me that I had basal cell carcinoma. It was very frightening so I wanted another opinion, and ultimately I went to a specialist in skin cancer. The diagnosis was a bit more complicated to come by, but finally it was diagnosed as squamous cell carcinoma.

With the kind of cancer I had, there are two ways to go—radiation or surgery. It was decided that radiation was not appropriate in my case, but the surgery that was planned would be quite disfiguring. I didn't want to do this and really scoured the world looking for alternatives, but finally I realized that I had no choice, and I had radical surgery. I had a completely bandaged nose for a year. As a matter of fact, I needed reconstructive surgery to give me a new nose, but it couldn't be done right away; they had to be sure that there was no sign of the cancer.

It took ten operations to completely rebuild a nose. I look different, but I'm happy that it wasn't more serious. Now, I wear big hats in the sun and the strongest sunscreen I can find, and swim only late in the day.

I think the most important lesson to be learned from my story—besides staying out of the sun—is that all of us should always seek expert dermatological guidance and advice if we see something questionable on our skin. In fact, I feel that one should always get opinions from more than one dermatologist. In my case, I spoke to several doctors, but none of them was trained to diagnose early skin cancer. By the time I got the treatment I needed, it had gone too far for a simple treatment, and I was faced with a long and complicated medical process.

Melanoma—A More Serious Problem

Like basal cell carcinoma, nearly all melanomas can be cured if detected early and treated promptly. However, there is no question that melanoma is a more serious and dangerous form of cancer. It is potentially fatal and must be treated immediately. The Skin Cancer Foundation identifies high-risk individuals as those who have:

· a family history of malignant melanoma
· had a malignant melanoma in the past
· unusual—dysplastic—moles (often larger than ¼ inch, irregular in shape, and multicolored)
· fair skin, light hair, and light eye color, and a tendency to sunburn easily and to tan with difficulty
· large brown moles at birth, or a record of painful or blistering sunburns, especially when young
· indoor occupations and outdoor recreational habits
· considerable outdoor exposure, especially while living in sunny regions

The Skin Cancer Foundation offers these warning signs:
Any one or more of these changes occurring in a new or existing pigmented (tan, brown) area of the skin, or in a mole, may indicate the presence of a malignant melanoma:

· *change in size:* especially sudden or continuous enlargement
· *change in color:* especially multiple shades of tan, brown, dark brown, black, the mixing of red, white, and blue; or the spreading of color from the edge into the surrounding skin
· *change in shape:* especially the developing of an irregular, notched border, which used to be regular
· *change in elevation:* especially the raising of a part of a pigmented area that used to be flat or only slightly elevated
· *change in surface:* especially scaliness, erosion, oozing, crusting, ulceration, or bleeding
· *change in surrounding skin:* especially redness; swelling; or the developing of colored blemishes next to, but not part of, the pigmented area
· *change in sensation:* especially itchiness, tenderness, or pain
· *change in consistency:* especially softening or hardening

The Skin Cancer Foundation suggests that everyone can reduce the risk of developing malignant melanoma. Here's how:

1. *Spend as little time as you can in the sun.* There is substantial evidence that sunlight is a causative factor for melanoma of the skin. Time in the sun should be reduced as much as possible. If you must be in the sun, avoid prolonged exposure between the hours of 10 A.M. and 2

P.M., when the sun is strongest; use a sunscreen rated SPF 15 or higher, and reapply it every 2 to 3 hours during long exposures or after swimming; wear a hat and tightly woven protective clothing; avoid getting sunburned; and do not try to get a "good tan."

2. *Examine your skin on a regular basis.* Begin with your face and scalp, step by step; look closely at your head, neck, shoulders, back, chest, arms, legs, etc. Become familiar with the differences between normal and dysplastic (changing) moles, and pay special attention to those moles that have unusual features. If any moles have changed, see a physician, preferably a specialist in diseases of the skin, right away.

3. *Select a physician for your skin care.* Have your skin checked at least once a year by this doctor. Sometimes, patients with dysplastic moles go through periods in which their moles are changing quickly and many new moles are appearing, such as in adolescence and pregnancy. During such episodes of increased mole activity, moles should be watched with special care and doctor visits increased to every three months.

4. *Get to know your skin.* Spend some time looking at your skin; learn what it looks like, where birthmarks and moles are located and what they look like. Don't forget the hard-to-see areas, especially the back, the scalp, between the buttocks, the genital area, and between your toes. Ask a friend or relative to help, and obtain a full-length mirror for self-examination.

5. *Changes in hormone balance may cause moles to change.* Extra medical check-ups are required during adolescence and pregnancy. The use of drugs, such as oral contraceptives or estrogens for treatment of menopausal symptoms, should be avoided for high-risk individuals, if possible.

Careful, regular self-examination, combined with frequent doctor visits, will detect skin changes early, and thus many changing moles will be removed before melanoma develops at all. Those few melanomas that do occur will almost always be discovered early in their course, at a time when they can be cured by surgery alone.

The Skin Cancer Foundation's List of Recommended Sunscreens

The Skin Cancer Foundation grants its seal of recommendation to sunscreen products of SPF 15 or greater that meet the Foundation's criteria as "aids in the prevention of sun-induced damage to the skin." As of

December 1988, the following products were approved by the Foundation's Photobiology Committee. New products are added to the list continually, and approved products are reevaluated on an annual basis.

Amway Corporation

Sunpacer Ultra Sunscreen Lotion SPF 15
Sunpacer Ultra Sunblock Stick SPF 15
Sunpacer Ultra Sunblock Creme SPF 30

Avon Products

Sunseekers SPF 24 Sunblock Lotion
Sunseekers "Children Formula" Sunblock Creme SPF 15

Carter-Wallace, Inc.

"Sea & Ski Block Out"
Ultra Sunblock Cream Lotion SPF 25 (waterproof)
Ultra Sunblock Clear Lotion SPF 20 (waterproof)
Ultra Sunblock Spray SPF 20 (waterproof)
Spray SPF 15 (waterproof)
Cream Lotion SPF 15 (waterproof)
Clear Lotion SPF 15 (waterproof)
Children's Sunblock Spray SPF 28 (waterproof)
Ultra Sunblock Clear Lotion SPF 28 (waterproof)
Ultra Sunblock Cream Lotion SPF 30 (waterproof)
Ultra Sunblock Spray SPF 28 (waterproof)
Children's Sunblock Lotion SPF 30 (waterproof)

Chesebrough-Pond's

Vaseline Lip Therapy SPF 15

Eclipse Laboratories

Skin Cancer Garde Sunblock Lotion SPF 33
Skin Cancer Garde Creme SPF 33
Child Garde Spray SPF 20
Child Garde Lotion SPF 30
Baby Garde SPF 25
Eclipse Lip and Face Protectant SPF 15
Total Eclipse Moisture Base Lotion SPF 15
Total Eclipse Alcohol Base Lotion SPF 15
Total Eclipse Sunblock Spray SPF 20
Total Eclipse PABA Free Lotion SPF 25

Estée Lauder

Estée Lauder Super Sunblock SPF 20
Estée Lauder Total Face Block SPF 25
Estée Lauder Waterworld Sunscreen SPF 15
Estée Lauder Waterworld Sunstick SPF 15

Giorgio, Inc.

Giorgio SPF 24 Superblock Lotion

Lancôme (Cosmair, Inc.)

Conquête du Soleil Barrière Solaire SPF 23
Conquête du Soleil Ecran Total Invisible SPF 15
Conquête du Soleil Ecran Solaire Waterproof SPF 15

Plough, Inc.

Coppertone Sunblock Lotion SPF 15
Coppertone Sunblock Lotion SPF 25
Coppertone Sunblock Lotion SPF 30+
Coppertone Noskote SPF 15
Coppertone Face SPF 15
SuperShade Sunblock Lotion SPF 15
SuperShade Sunblock Lotion SPF 25
SuperShade Sunblock Lotion SPF 30+
SuperShade Sunblock Stick SPF 25
Water Babies Sunblock Lotion SPF 15
Water Babies Sunblock Creme SPF 25
Water Babies Sunblock Lotion SPF 30+
Tropical Blend Lotion SPF 15

Richardson-Vicks

Bain de Soleil Ultra Sun Block Creme SPF 30
Bain de Soleil Ultra Sun Block Creme SPF 15
Bain de Soleil Under Eye Protector SPF 15
Bain de Soleil Ultra Sun Block Lip Balm SPF 15
Bain de Soleil Moisture Tanning Face Creme SPF 15

Westwood Pharmaceuticals

Presun 39 Creamy Sunscreen
Presun for Kids SPF 29
Presun 29 Sensitive Skin Sunscreen

Presun 15 Sensitive Skin Sunscreen
Presun 15 Creamy Sunscreen
Presun 15 Lotion Sunscreen
Presun 15 Facial Stick
Presun 15 Lip Protector
Presun 15 Facial Sunscreen

Within this list are many different kinds of products. Chesebrough-Pond's Vaseline has a lip product, for example. Bain de Soleil has several sunscreens, including one called Moisture Tanning Face Creme, said by the company to be a noncomedegenic moisturizing product, to be less greasy, and to work well under makeup. Westwood has several different formulas, including one for sensitive skin.

There are really very few reasons why most of you cannot find a sunscreen product that works for your skin. Considering the risks of skin cancer, not to mention premature aging and sun-induced wrinkling and age spots, it seems like a small investment of time and money to find one that makes you happy and protects your skin.

For more information about skin cancer and its prevention or an updated list of the Skin Cancer Foundation's list of recommended sunscreens, write to:

> The Skin Cancer Foundation
> P.O. Box 561
> New York, NY 10156

FOUR

Designing Your Own Skin Care Program: Knowing What to Buy and How to Use It

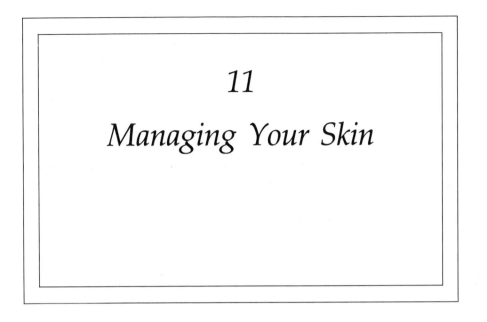

11

Managing Your Skin

I know that there are women out there with perfectly managed skin and tried-and-true skin care rituals. You may be one of them, but in case you're not, see if you identify with any of the three major types with mismanaged skin:

1. women who do the wrong thing
2. women who don't do enough
3. women who do too much

Women Who Do the Wrong Thing

Type One: Comedegenic Dora Dora knows that she has oily, acne-prone skin, but she doesn't deal with it realistically. She continues to risk cosmetic acne with comedegenic products, and then, when she has a flare-up, instead of visiting a dermatologist or even trying some of the over-the-counter drying acne medications, Dora keeps trying to cure her acne breakouts with cosmetic products such as scrubs and toners and cleansers. Sometimes they work; more often they don't.

Type Two: Overmoisturized Marilyn Marilyn's skin is on the dry side, at least some of the time. But much of the time, it is combination skin. Her T-zone is mildly oily and the rest of her face is normal. However, Marilyn has read all the ads about anti-aging products and wants to avoid wrinkles and consequently has used so much moisturizer that her skin is dull and caked-looking. Marilyn makes the mistake of thinking that it is getting dryer and instead of washing it with soap and water, she quickly purchases an extrarich and oily cleanser. Marilyn's skin would be beautiful if she knew what to do, but she doesn't.

Type Three: Sweet Dishpan Sue We've all heard about dishpan hands. Well, Sweet Sue has dishpan face. Sweet Sue, who has mildly oily skin, is afraid of acne, and she seriously believes that if she just keeps her skin clean enough and dry enough nothing bad can happen to her. So she uses a drying soap and scrubbing grains and a clay mask. Then when she is so shiny and dry that she feels that a smile will make her face crack, she faces the world—without a moisturizer.

Women Who Don't Do Enough

Type One: Soap-and-Water Sally We all know women like this—no lotions or potions for them. They believe in doing what comes naturally. Only good old soap and water. They often don't even use sunscreens. The only problem is that typically this woman desperately needs a moisturizer. While her tan is getting deeper and deeper, her skin is getting dryer and dryer.

Type Two: Cover-It-Over Candy Unlike   Soap-and-Water   Sally, Candy doesn't have a philosophy about her skin. She just doesn't want to take the time to deal with her skin. Some of her pores are clogged, and her complexion is muddy. One of these days, she tells herself, she'll get herself a facial and get her pores cleaned. But she has so many other good uses for the money. In the meantime, she uses makeup to cover her whiteheads.

Women Who Do Too Much

Type One: Overzealous Zeena Zeena wants desperately to do what's right for her skin, so she does what's right, and she does what's right. And a few hours later, she does it again. Then, worried that she may not have done it right, or might not have used the right products, she goes to the store, returns home with a new product line, and does it once again.

She has washed her face with almost all the soaps or cleansers advertised; she has scrubbed with everything from apples to plastic; she has splashed, rinsed, patted, and sprayed her face with every toner, refresher, astringent, clarifier, and spritzer manufactured. Wrinkle control? Zeena knows about wrinkle control. She has used collagen, elastin, hormone creams, placenta creams, cell-renewal creams, firming serums, cellular ampules, not to mention throat cream, eye cream, microsomes, liposomes, niosomes, and, once on the advice of her hairdresser, Preparation H.

She has had her skin analyzed and typed by salespeople, color consultants, computer printouts, and salon managers. She has had so many facials that it's a miracle she has any skin left. In short, she has been scrubbed like a pot.

Zeena now has a new problem. Her skin is so sensitive that she is zealously on the search for new products, any products, that won't make her itch, burn, or tingle.

Managing Your Skin the Right Way, Regardless of Skin Type

1. Determine Your Skin Type and Develop a Realistic Skin Care Program If you are a skin care user, and you have skin that is too dry or too oily, scaling or breaking out, then there is every possibility that you are using the wrong products and doing the wrong thing. Women who do the wrong thing for their skin are most often misinformed about their skin type. If you have a history of taking care of your skin and still having complexion problems, your first skin care priority is to accurately determine your *current* skin type, which may be different from what you believe, and then to develop a carefully thought-out and realistic skin care program based on your actual needs.

2. Develop a Simple Skin Care Program That Is Easy to Follow It's important to develop a simple skin care routine that can be easily incorporated into your daily routine. If grooming concerns are not priorities in your life, and you have a tendency to neglect your skin, you should never purchase products for a complicated skin care program because chances are that most, if not all, of those products will end up unused in a drawer somewhere.

If you are a woman who doesn't do enough for her skin, you, more than any other type, need to find a small group of products that makes you happy. Choose products that are easily replaced and make certain your skin care shopping is done in a spot that is conveniently located.

If skin care is not a major concern in your life, for the most part you should also choose products that are moderately priced. Otherwise, when the time comes to replace them, there is a very good possibility that you will resist doing so and think of more important things to do with your money.

3. Less Is More No matter what your skin type is, the cardinal rule is to keep your skin care routine simple and not become a skin care junkie. Complicated chemical formulas combined with excessive washing, scrubbing, and massaging can traumatize even the healthiest skin. It's human and understandable to strive for perfection, but, as far as skin care is concerned, this tendency to overdo can create major complexion problems. Skin is intrinsically fragile and delicate. It has a definite pH of its own and it is easily irritated, chapped, chafed, and sensitized. Cosmetic products, including both makeup and skin care, are composed of thousands of chemical combinations. Because they have different acid and alkaline values, they automatically tend to alter an individual's pH.

Often the woman who has the most problems with her skin is the woman who is doing it all, and too often. She may know her skin type, but so many different chemical combinations have been applied to her skin that she has made it irritable and supersensitive. All the handling and scrubbing has only exacerbated the condition.

Several dermatologists have talked to me about this particular type of skin care consumer. Typically, she is someone who wants to do the right thing for her skin, but she is just overzealous in her care. Incidentally, at least one study shows that this type of consumer is the one who ends up with the most sensitive skin. Obviously, this type of skin presents a real problem because often a vicious cycle is set up in which the skin becomes more and more reactive and the consumer becomes more and more determined to find something that works for her skin.

Designing Your Skin Care Program—Let Your Skin Type Be Your Guide

Whether your skin is dry, oily, normal, or combination, you need products that are specifically designed for you. There is no one perfect soap, perfect cleanser, or perfect moisturizer. You have to design your own program. Your skin type is the first consideration. But remember: *Skin type changes as one ages, and it should be reevaluated every six months.*

General Guidelines for Dry Skin

If you have dry skin, your basic guidelines are very simple:

· Be careful not to strip the skin of natural oils with harsh cleansing routines.

- Keep your skin moist by wearing an appropriate moisturizer at all times.
- Avoid further drying and premature aging by using a sunscreen with SPF 15 whenever you are going to be exposed to ultraviolet rays.
- Buy products with ingredients that are nondrying and nonirritating to your skin.

General Guidelines for Oily or Acne-Prone Skin

Oily skin is not as simple to manage as dry skin. For one thing, there are so many degrees of oiliness. Mildly oily skin with rare breakouts is quite different from very oily skin with frequent breakouts. Women with very oily, acne-prone skin need to be particularly careful about what they use on their faces. These women should also realize that even if they have only a few pimples or comedones, they are experiencing an acne-type breakout. This is a medical condition and should not be treated with *cosmetic* facial preparation without a dermatologist's advice. There are several very effective over-the-counter *drug* preparations for the treatment of acne. Here is advice for women with oily skin:

- Avoid comedegenic ingredients and don't contribute to your oily skin by using products that will clog your pores or make your skin even oilier.
- Don't overreact to your oily skin by irritating it with overly harsh washing and scrubbing techniques.
- Do establish a sensible cleansing technique that keeps your skin free of oils.
- Don't disregard or minimize acne breakouts or attempt to self-treat acne with cosmetic products.
- Wear a noncomedegenic sunscreen with an appropriate SPF whenever you are exposed to the sun.
- Do treat acne by getting appropriate *medical* guidance and advice.

General Guidelines for Normal Skin

Keep your skin normal by not taking advantage of your genetic good fortune. Normal skin requires very little care. All you have to do is stay in the middle, avoiding products that are too extreme.

· Do develop an uncomplicated daily cleansing routine.
· Don't smother your skin with unnecessarily heavy moisturizers and creams.
· Do apply a sunscreen with the appropriate SPF whenever you are going to be exposed to solar radiation.
· Don't buy products with ingredients that are either too oily or too drying.

General Guidelines for Combination Skin

Because you have two skin types at once, you need a program that works for both parts of your face.

· Do develop an effective cleansing program for your entire face.
· Do keep your T-zone free of unnecessary oils.
· Moisturize only the dry parts of your skin.
· Do apply a noncomedegenic sunscreen with the appropriate SPF whenever you are going to be exposed to solar radiation.
· Products that are applied in the T-zone should not include ingredients that will clog the pores.

All Skin Types—Buying What's Right and Rejecting What's Wrong

When buying a skin care product, the first thing to do is to look carefully at what the package says. Here are some clues to help you translate the terminology. If the package says:

"Dry or mature skin"—You can be fairly certain that the product has emollients and other moisturizing ingredients. Products that say they are best for dry or mature skin are absolutely off limits for women with oily or oily, acne-prone skin. They may also be too "rich" for women with normal or combination-type skin.

"Oily skin"—These products usually include ingredients that will dry the skin or soak up oils. They will almost always be too drying for women with dry or mature skin, and will often be too drying for women with

normal skin. Most of the time, combination-type skin can use these products in the T-zone. However, some products, even though they specify "oily skin," contain ingredients that are occasionally comedegenic.

"*Noncomedegenic*"—This is a relatively new term, used on labels for many of the oily skin programs. Even though there are no absolute standards, most manufacturers make a real attempt to exclude comedegenic ingredients from these products. As one might expect, products for oily skin are often drying, which is what one wants for oily, acne-prone skin. They may, however, be a bit too drying for women with normal-to-oily skin.

"*Normal*" or "*combination*" *skin*—These products can be confusing because many women have skin that would more aptly be described as normal-to-dry or normal-to-oily. What this means is that if your skin tends to be a *little* too oily, these products are sometimes a *little* too rich. Only the ingredients can help you decide.

"*Normal-to-oily skin*"—These products are sometimes best suited for skin that is truly normal; at other times, for skin that is slightly oily. You have to check the ingredients.

"*Normal-to-dry skin*"—These products are most likely to have emollients. If you have combination skin, they are probably not suited for your T-zone.

"*All skin types*"—These are the most confusing words and, in my opinion, the most likely to be misleading. Always check the ingredients before purchasing these products, particularly if you have oily skin.

Reading the Ingredients Label The only sure way to know what kinds of ingredients are in a product is to read the ingredients label. Because the ingredients have to be listed in descending order of predominance, the first five or six listed will give you a fairly clear picture of whether or not the product is right for your skin.

The ingredients further down on the list are not as significant in determining whether the product is best for oily or dry skin. However, they still tell you what's in the product, and if you have either acne- or allergic-type breakouts, sometimes it is one of these less important ingredients that can be irritating for you.

Typically, the last few ingredients listed on the label are preservatives, color additives, and fragrance.

Choosing Ingredients for Dry Skin

Because you want to replace oils and prevent moisture loss, you want to avoid ingredients that are drying or that absorb oils. Some of these are: alcohol, witch hazel, recorcinol, salicylic acid, kaolin, clay, talc, and magnesium aluminum silicate.

Choose products with emollients, moisturizing agents, fatty alcohols, and protectants. Here's a list:

acetylated lanolin alcohol

allantoin

amino acids (There are twenty-two amino acids, including glycine, alanine, valine, leucine, isoleucine, serine, threonine, cysteine, glutamine acid, arganine.)

cetyl alcohol (a fatty alcohol)

collagen

cyclomethicone

dimethicone

hyaluronic acid

hydrolyzed animal protein

isopropyl myristate

isopropyl palmitate

isostearic acid

lanolin

lanolin alcohol

linoleic acid

mineral oil

mucopolysaccharides

myristic acid

myristyl myristate

natural moisturizing factors

petrolatum

squalane

stearic acid

stearyl alcohol (a fatty alcohol)

triglycerides

urea

vegetable oils

Choosing Ingredients for Oily Skin

Some ingredients rarely, if ever, cause acne-type breakouts. When a product is formulated specifically for oily or acne-prone skin, and the manufacturer wants to make it clear that it doesn't think anything in the product will cause acne, the word that is most frequently used is non-comedegenic.

Because the most frequent tests of comedegenic or noncomedegenic are done on rabbits' ears, there is no certainty that all women will respond the same way. The phrase "noncomedegenic" essentially means that the ingredients within the product are not likely to cause acne or pimples, but there are no guarantees.

When skin care products, or any other cosmetic product, produce comedones, the result is called cosmetic acne. For some women, all this amounts to is a few pimples, but there are others who have experienced truly unnecessary grief as a result of applying the wrong substances to their faces.

A Scary Story About What Can Happen If You Use Skin Care Products That Are Not Right for Your Skin This is an unfortunate story of high-pressure selling, comedegenic skin care products, an unsuspecting customer, and severe cosmetic acne, and although I don't normally like to use this kind of scare technique to emphasize the importance of proper skin care, it is a true story and it's worth repeating.

This story began in 1982, when a young model, recently signed by one of the most prestigious New York modeling agencies, decided that she wanted to make certain that she was getting the best care for her skin and went to a store where she was sold a line of well-known, as well as expensive, skin care products, including cleansers and astringents, by a white-coated "specialist." She took the products home, used them, and broke out. When she returned to the store to consult the "specialist," she was told that it was just a temporary phase and was encouraged to buy more products, which she did. But she still had problems. This time when she returned, the specialist consulted an "advisor" in the company's main office. The "advisor" suggested buying more products. All in all, she spent over $400. Within eight months of following this "professional" advice, the model's face was so permanently pitted by acne scars that it was determined that not even dermabrasion could get rid of them.

Ultimately the model sued, and in the trial it was revealed that the products sold to the model had contained comedegenic ingredients that could cause acne flare-ups; these ingredients were later removed from the products. The model's attorneys argued that the products had been slickly marketed in a way that was calculated to mislead and that the company was negligent in failing to list ingredients and post warnings and instructions on the products. The company countered by saying that the model should have ignored the "expert" advice and stopped using the product.

Because the woman's career had been devastated, her loss was substantial, and the court found that the skin care company's negligent manufacture, marketing, and instruction were at fault, and, in 1987, awarded the woman $2 million for her lost earnings and career as well as for her suffering and emotional distress. The case is currently on appeal and the amount is expected to be reduced.

I doubt if the manufacturer wanted to cause so much distress, but it seems apparent that the products were marketed with comedegenic ingredients and that the "expert" was a salesperson who failed to correctly evaluate the young woman's skin when recommending products, and didn't understand or recognize cosmetic acne.

Granted, this case is an extreme. However, I've interviewed hundreds of women and I'm always amazed at how many of them, even older women with dry skin, have had a breakout that they associated with using a cosmetic product that was too oily.

Most cases of cosmetic acne will occur within a few weeks of using a product, but in some instances it can take longer.

Potentially Comedegenic Ingredients There is some disagreement among researchers as to which ingredients are most likely to be comedegenic, and not everyone agrees. Here is a list of ingredients that have been cited by one or more dermatologists as potentially comedegenic:

acetylated lanolin	isodecyl oleate (slight)
acetylated lanolin alcohol	isopropyl isostearate
butyl stearate	isopropyl lanolate
castor oil (slight)	isopropyl linoleate
cetyl alcohol	isopropyl myristate
cocoa butter	isopropyl palmitate
corn oil (slight)	isostearyl neopentanoate
decyl oleate	lanolin
ethoxylated lanolin	lanolin acid
glyceryl monostearate	lanolin alcohol
grape seed oil	lanolin oil (slight)
hydroxypropyl cellulose	laureth 4
isocetyl stearate (slight)	lauryl alcohol (slight)

mineral oil (slight)	peach kernel oil
myristyl alcohol (slight)	PPG-2 myristyl propionate
myristyl lactate	propylene glycol isostearate
myristyl myristate	propylene glycol monostearate
octyl palmitate	stearic acid
oleic acid	stearyl alcohol
oleyl alcohol	sweet almond oil

Designed for Oily Skin Products that are intended for oily, acne-prone skin are either formulated without oils or formulated with oils that are not considered overwhelmingly comedegenic. There is some disagreement over this. Consequently, if you look at the labels of some oily-skin products, you will find ingredients that one set of experts okayed and that another set of experts believe to be comedegenic. Reasonably safe moisturizing ingredients for oily skin are humectants such as propylene glycol or glycerin. Oily-skin products tend to be high in alcohol, which is drying, and they sometimes include an ingredient that absorbs oils, such as magnesium aluminum silicate or talc.

Choosing Ingredients for Sensitive or Allergy-Prone Skin

It is nearly impossible to come up with a definitive list of all the ingredients that might prove to be potentially irritating. No two women are precisely the same. Mineral oil, for example, is one of the most popular cosmetics ingredients, and very few women are allergic to it. Yet I've received letters from two women saying that they are allergic to mineral oil and asking me to mention this potential problem. It would appear that there is no guarantee that a specific ingredient will never be an irritant.

However, in the last few years it seems to me that cosmetics manufacturers have made efforts to reduce the number of irritants in cosmetics and skin care products. Also, they seem to have made real attempts to do away with confusing language such as the word hypoallergenic. Hypo means "less than," and the word hypoallergenic tells the consumer that the manufacturer believes the product has fewer allergens than other products. There are no federal regulations defining allergens, nor are there any guidelines, so the "hypoallergenic" has little real meaning.

Here are some of the ingredients most frequently cited as potential irritants.

Fragrance—Fragrance is probably the most common allergen in skin care products.

Coal tar dyes—There are many fewer coal tar dyes in skin care products than in other types of cosmetics. Nonetheless, one still sees them, particularly in toners. A fair number of women react badly to these, particularly when they are used around the eyes, since the dye can cause stinging and burning. If a moisturizer contains a coal tar dye, it is advisable to not apply it near the eyes. Technically, coal tars are prohibited from being included in products that are meant for use in the eye area.

Lanolin—Lanolin is frequently mentioned as an allergen.

Preservatives—Skin care products certainly need preservatives. Nonetheless, they can sometimes be irritating. Some of the most common preservatives used in skin care products include: benzyl paraben, butyl paraben, ethyl paraben, quaternium-15, imidazolidinyl urea, sodium dehydroacetate, glutaral, sodium borate, methylchloroisothiazolinone, methylisothiazolinone.

Detergent ingredients—Many products, including astringents, soaps, and some creams, contain detergents. The ones most often mentioned seem to be sodium laurel sulfate and laureth 4.

Certain oils—The following oils are mentioned as being irritants: cinnamon, clove, eucalyptus, bitter almond, lemon, orange, wintergreen, and bergamot.

Some "natural" ingredients—Some of the natural ingredients derived from plant sources are sometimes mentioned as allergens. Also, some women are sensitive to vitamin E, particularly when it is applied directly to the skin, as opposed to being included in a cream or lotion base.

Women with very sensitive skin should also avoid abrasives such as rough grains or ground seeds or nuts. These include natural ingredients such as ground apricot kernel as well as polyethylene granules.

Nonprescription Skin Protectants If you have sensitive skin, you should be aware of an FDA list of ingredients classified as safe and effective nonprescription skin protectants. When you see a skin protection claim, one or more of these ingredients may be included:

allantoin	kaolin
calamine	petrolatum
cocoa butter	shark liver oil
dimethicone	zinc oxide
glycerin	

Choosing Ingredients for Normal Skin

Normal-to-Oily Normal Skin Your skin is definitely too oily to use rich moisturizers in which the ingredients are heavily weighed in favor of emollients such as lanolin or esters such as myristyl myristate. But your skin may not be so oily that it won't become parched looking if you use very drying products formulated for very oily skin. These include "moisturizers" that are mostly alcohol and astringents with drying ingredients such as resorcinol or salycilic acid.

Normal-to-Dry Normal Skin Your skin is too dry to use the drying products formulated for oily skin, but your skin may not be so dry or mature that you can safely apply any and all moisturizers and anti-aging products without risking pimples, clogged pores, or little white bumps under your skin. Choose moisturizing ingredients that are less likely to be comedegenic, such as petrolatum, mineral oil, propylene glycol, and glycerin.

Combination Skin

Choose your ingredients depending upon how oily you are in your T-zone and how dry you are on your cheeks and sides of your face.

Women who get clogged pores and pimples in their T-zone should avoid the same ingredients as women with oily skin. But that doesn't mean that you can use drying products such as alcohol-based moisturizers and cleansers on your non-T-zone areas. Makeup and skin care products tend to slide across one's face, so avoid comedegenic moisturizers as well as foundation makeup.

12

How to Wash Your Face and What to Wash It With

Most of us wash our faces too often. Some of us don't wash them often enough. And most of us don't pay enough attention to what we wash them with. As a matter of fact, most cases of mismanaged skin start in the cleansing process. Cleansing products, which are by definition filled with soaps, abrasives, and detergents, combined with cleansing practices that often involve very hot water and too much rub-a-dub-dub have the potential to damage the skin.

Cleansing Tips, Hints, and Cautions for All Skin Types

Daily Cleansing Routines

1. *Remove all traces of old makeup before going to bed.*
   Nothing clogs pores or creates complexion problems more than the

remains of yesterday's glamorous face. Shadow, blusher, and foundation can leave oily deposits in the pores.

2. *Wash your face gently and quickly.*

Zealously rubbing at the face with soap and water causes too much friction. This can create inflammation, irritate pores, and is generally destructive to sensible skin care. Remember, blackheads are not caused by dirt and rubbing does not make them disappear.

3. *Always rinse well and remove all traces of soap.*

When you rinse your skin, splash your face at least fifteen times to make sure there are no signs of soap left on your face.

4. *Don't use water that is too hot, too cold, or too hard.*

Hot water can damage capillaries. Dermatologists advise against using water that is either too hot or too cold. Lukewarm water is best for your skin. Where you live can also make a difference in how you wash your face. Women who live in a hard-water area may need to double or triple their rinse time. Some women prefer to use bottled water for the final rinse.

5. *Don't wash your face more than is necessary.*

Let your skin type be your guide on this one, and don't dry out your face by washing it more than is appropriate.

Rules for Using Exfoliating Scrubs

1. *Don't get obsessive!*

Women sometimes cause havoc with their skin by going overboard with abrasive cleansers. They think that they can scrub away pimples and other complexion problems. Not so. It's the other way around—heavy duty scrubbing can cause pimples.

Whether you are using an abrasive sponge such as a Buf-Puf or a creamy scrub cleanser such as Adrien Arpel's Honey and Almond Scrub, the trick is to remember that less is more effective.

Scrubs should be used on clean, *wet* skin. Moisten your face with warm water first; that softens the top layer and prepares it for the scrub. Then, using a circular motion, massage gently. Don't spend more than a few seconds on any one area of your face. The entire procedure should be finished in *less than thirty seconds.* Don't use any form of scrub or abrasive in the eye area.

Overly energetic long-term use of harsh abrasives can ultimately damage the skin and cause problems later.

If you are using an abrasive cleanser, rinse it off in tepid water. Keep splashing until it is entirely rinsed off. Then pat dry.

2. Don't use a scrub cleanser too often.

If you have oily skin, two or three times a week is more than enough. If you have dry skin, once a week is all you need.

3. Don't use two types of abrasives or an abrasive and another cleanser simultaneously.

Women sometimes make the mistake of trying to apply abrasive grain-type cleansers with equally abrasive sponges and/or loofas. You also shouldn't use an abrasive in combination with another cleansing product. This combining of abrasives can result in seriously irritated skin.

4. Don't use scrub products near the eyes.

No scrubs or any forms of abrasives should be used anywhere in the eye area. The skin is much too delicate.

Black women should take special care to not injure their skins with harsh ingredients because of possible scarring and pigment changes. Some abrasive ingredients are harder than others and, hence, more potentially damaging. Some examples of extreme hardness include apricot seeds, various nut shells, and silica. If the particle is small enough, it can compensate for this hardness, but women of all skin types should always use a light touch and low energy when employing these ingredients. *And, if it hurts, stop using it!*

To Steam or Not to Steam

Steaming your skin is a time-honored method of deep cleaning and getting the "gunk" out of the pores. As a matter of fact, it is one of my favorites. However, I should tell you that most dermatologists and skin care experts would advise against it, saying that the hot water is bad for your skin because it is potentially drying and can damage capillaries, causing little red lines in your skin. Dermatologists also remind us that heat and humidity can induce an acne-type flare-up. So if the capillaries on your nose or cheeks are fragile, and you are acne-prone, then steaming is a definite No.

Rules for Using Deep-Cleansing Masks

1. Keep them away from the area around the eyes. They are too drying for the delicate skin found in the eye area.
2. Follow instructions and don't let a cleansing mask stay on your face any longer than instructed.

Some Words of Caution About Using Astringents and Toners

When choosing astringents and toners, read the ingredients label carefully. Some are medicated and include ingredients such as resorcinol and salicylic acid. In appropriate concentrations, these are anti-acne drugs and can be very drying for normal skin. Alcohol toners by definition are drying, but many include additional ingredients such as sodium borate, camphor, and menthol; these make the product even more drying as well as potentially irritating.

Many, if not all, toners contain coal tar dyes. These colors can be comedegenic and/or irritating. Many toners contain fragrance; this can also be an irritant. Toners should not be applied near the eyes.

A toner or astringent product is not advisable for anyone using Retin-A. Again, it can be too drying.

Black women should note that resorcinol, which is included in some astringent products, can leave a brownish scale.

Removing Cream Cleansers—Do Not Tissue Off!

Whenever you remove cream cleansers, use a wet washcloth. *Never tissue off a cleansing cream or any other skin care or cosmetic product!* Here's why: Tissues, as well as other paper products, are made from wood pulp and are irritating to the skin. So, no matter what the instructions say, don't use tissues.

General Cleansing Guidelines for Women with Dry Skin

The first rule of caring for dry skin is very simple: Don't use anything that is going to dry it out further. Because many products marketed as soaps or cleansers are intrinsically drying, choose your cleansing products carefully. Many soaps, for example, have an alkaline pH; this means that they can have a drying effect. And cleansing creams often contain ingredients that can be drying or irritating if they are not removed properly. That's why the consumer with dry skin receives confusing information about how to clean her face and that's also why skin care companies promote two or more different kinds of cleansers for dry skin.

Some skin care companies say soaps and detergents are drying and promote cream cleansers that they say will not be drying, but that will lubricate. The only problem with most of these cream cleansers is that, more often than not, they include a soap or detergent-type ingredient, which is also drying. That's why anyone using a cream cleanser is advised to remove it thoroughly. If you visit the department store cosmetics counter, chances are you will have a dialogue that goes something like this:

Ms. Dry Skin: "I want to know how to cleanse my face."

Cosmetics salesperson: "Let's see. What skin type do you have?"

Ms. Dry Skin: "Dry . . . very dry. I don't know what to do."

Cosmetics salesperson: "What are you presently using to wash your face?"

Ms. Dry Skin: "Soap and water."

Cosmetics salesperson: "My dear, that is a real No-no. That's one of the reasons your skin is so dry. Let me show you what you should be using."

At this point, your cosmetics salesperson reaches into his/her supplies and appears with a cleansing cream tester, which he/she applies to the back of your hand, rubs it lightly into the skin, and then removes it with a tissue.

Cosmetics salesperson: "See how smooth and soft your skin feels now."

Ms. Dry Skin: "You're right! It feels great. I'll take it."

Cosmetics salesperson: "Now, do you know how to use this? Twice a day, morning and evening, massage a small amount of cleanser onto your skin. Tissue or rinse off. Then follow up with this toning lotion, which is especially formulated for dry skin, to remove dirt and whatever else is left on your skin."

Ms. Dry Skin: "I have to use something after the cleanser?"

Cosmetics salesperson: "Oh yes, this is very important. If you don't use a toner, you can end up with clogged pores."

Clogged pores are the reason some skin care companies have almost abandoned the heavy cream-cleanser, except as a makeup remover, and are concentrating instead on marketing the soap or detergent-type cleansing product, packaged in a tube or some other container for the consumer with dry skin. Sometimes these are called gels or foams. One cannot often tell whether it is a soap or a detergent except by reading the promotional copy or listening to the salesperson. If it is a detergent, the copy will say something like, "Contains no harsh soaps." If it is a soap, the copy will say something like, "Contains no harsh detergents."

These products are not cream cleansers, although they may contain some emollients. Whether they are soaps or detergents, they are very expensive cleansing products.

The fact is that the woman with dry skin *should* avoid stripping the oils from her skin with harsh cleansing products.

The solution, however, is not using a cream cleanser.

Your Dry Skin Care Routine

How Often to Cleanse Your Face If you truly have dry or mature skin, you shouldn't have to wash your face with a cleansing product more than once a day—in the evening, when you remove your makeup.

Forget all your cleansers and soaps in the morning. All you need is water. Just wash your face with a warm washcloth. Use the water and the washcloth to wipe away any dead skin cells and oily debris. Then splash your face with water—at least twenty splashes—and apply your moisturizer. You can repeat this process as many times during the day as you want. I suggest doing it at least twice daily to get moisture back into the cells.

Before Going to Bed
Step 1. If you have been wearing heavy makeup and must use a cream to remove it, apply a layer of the cream (some products are listed on page 209) and lightly massage it in. Use lukewarm water and a wet washcloth

to remove oil and makeup. If you are wearing little or no makeup, go directly to:

Step 2. Wash your face as follows: Using your cleansing product, with your fingertips or a soft washcloth work up a lather on your face. Use gentle circular motions and do it as quickly as possible; it shouldn't take more than fifteen to twenty seconds. Splash your face to remove soap and wipe off the excess with a wet washcloth.

Step 3. Rinse your face well, splashing an additional twenty handfuls of water onto your face.

Step 4. Pat lightly with a soft towel, but don't dry completely.

Step 5. Apply a heavy moisturizer on your face.

When You Wake Up

Step 1. Splash your face at least five times with lukewarm water.

Step 2. Wash your face with a lukewarm washcloth (no soap). The mildly abrasive effect of the washcloth and the warm water should wipe away the remains of old moisturizer and any superficial dirt that has accumulated.

Step 3. Splash your face an additional twenty times with lukewarm water.

Step 4. Pat with soft towel, but don't dry completely.

Step 5. Apply a moisturizer.

Step 6. Use a sunscreen with an appropriate SPF whenever you are exposed to ultraviolet light.

Once a week: Scrub, with mild, gentle Buf-Puf, or cornmeal. Moisturizing facial mask: see page 128 for a list of products.

Choosing Your Basic Cleansing Product

In my opinion, if you have dry skin, your basic cleansing product should be a soap or a detergent cleanser that has added emolliency. Some choices are:

pHisoderm Liquid (dry skin formula)—pHisoderm Liquid is pH-adjusted. It contains a detergent as well as emollients (petrolatum and lanolin alcohol) and does an excellent job of removing dirt and makeup.

Alpha Keri Moisturizing Soap—Alpha Keri is a nondetergent bar soap that contains emollients, including lanolin oil and mineral oil.

Neutrogena Dry Skin Soap—This is a pH-adjusted soap that includes emollients as well as glycerin, a humectant.

Aveeno Cleansing Bar (dry skin formula)—Aveeno is soap-free. It contains a mild surfactant as well as oatmeal, emollients, and glycerin.

Dove—This is a detergent bar that includes emollients; it has a deserved reputation for mildness.

Removing Makeup with Cleansing Cream If you use little or no makeup, you rarely, if ever, have any need for a heavy cream-cleanser. However, makeup, particularly those products designed for dry skin, is mostly oil-based, and if you wear a lot of it, you sometimes need an oily substance to get it off your face.

There are several very good, very inexpensive options. These are products of simple formulations with few unnecessary ingredients and are about as nonirritating as possible.

· Albolene (scented and unscented)
  Advantages: can be used effectively on makeup that is extremely difficult to remove, including stage makeup; inexpensive
  Disadvantages: somewhat greasy; contains ceresin, which in rare instances may cause an allergic dermatitis. (The scented formula contains a fragrance to which some women may be allergic.)
· Baby oil
  Advantages: inexpensive and effective; one simple ingredient, mineral oil, plus fragrance
  Disadvantage: contains fragrance to which some women may be sensitive
· Crisco
  Advantages: inexpensive and effective
  Disadvantages: aesthetically unappealing; potentially comedegenic
· Nivea Oil
  Advantages: inexpensive; also a moisturizer
  Disadvantage: somewhat greasy
· Pond's Essential Cleansing Cream
  Advantages: inexpensive and effective
  Disadvantage: a true cleansing cream and should be thoroughly removed

Some women are not comfortable using inexpensive skin care products, no matter how effective they may be. If you are one of these women, there are, of course, many cleansing creams designed to remove makeup from dry skin. Two that I have liked over the years are Chanel's Melting Cleanser and Adrien Arpel's Coconut Cleanser.

Dry Skin and Toning Lotions—Do You Need One?

Some skin care companies market toners that are specifically designed for women with dry skin. Toners meant for dry skin typically do not include alcohol, which is drying.

Normally, women with dry skin have little need for a toning lotion. But there are times when even a woman with dry skin may want to use a toning lotion, in her T-zone *only*. For example, after removing heavy makeup with a heavy cream-cleanser, a dry-skin toning lotion can sometimes be used to wipe away any residue as well as the oily film. This process is not necessary if you are using a soap-type product. And in the summer, even women with dry skin can sometimes perspire and become a little oily in the T-zone area.

Women with dry skin should not use a toner after a soap-and-water cleansing.

Women with very dry, mature, or sensitive skin rarely, if ever, need a toning lotion.

If you have pores in the T-zone area that are becoming clogged and need the extra attention of a toner, then chances are that you *do not* have dry skin and, instead, have combination skin and should be treating it accordingly.

Cleansing Masks and Dry Skin

If you have true dry skin, with small or nonvisible pores, then you don't need to use a clay or "deep cleaning" mask. As the clay is drying, it can actually be absorbing moisture from your skin. But, if you have pores that get clogged and need cleaning, you probably have combination skin.

Most vinyl peel-off masks are not suitable for dry skin, either. Peel-off masks can damage capillaries or irritate sensitive skin.

Using a Scrub—If You Have Dry or Mature Skin

There has been a good deal of publicity over the years that stressed the use of scrubs for oily skin. This has tended to make the average woman with dry or mature skin assume that she doesn't need to use a scrub on her face. This is unfortunate, because the woman with dry or mature skin often realizes the best results from regularly exfoliating her skin, on a weekly basis, with an abrasive cleansing product.

Use a scrub once a week, but as much as possible choose a product that doesn't irritate your dry skin. My favorite is a Buf-Puf (gentle), which has no additional ingredients. Finely ground cornmeal is another inexpensive solution. Stay away from scrub cleansers that have additional cleansing ingredients such as detergents, soaps, or surfactants. If you want to buy a cosmetic preparation, look for scrub cleansers that have creams or oils. You can make any scrub less abrasive by thinning it with an emollient.

Before using the scrub, splash your face with tepid water at least ten times to give the skin a chance to soften naturally.

Don't use a scrub more than once a week. Remember, no more than thirty seconds of circular motion for the entire face. Keep the motion gentle. Don't irritate the skin.

Cleansing Guidelines for Dry, Sensitive Skin

If you have dry skin that is also sensitive, you can follow most of the dry-skin suggestions. However, your skin is probably too sensitive for scrub products, toners, or astringents at any time. Keep your cleansing products simple; several dermatologists suggest Dove as a mild soap. More than those who have any other skin type, you should avoid hot water or harsh cleansing techniques. Avoid products that include fragrance or other well-known irritants. As much as possible, try to wash your face at least half an hour before you put on clothing, particularly woolens. Make certain your face is dry before you go outdoors, and always rinse off all traces of soap.

Cleansing Guidelines for Oily Skin

The first rule of caring for oily skin is: Don't use anything that is going to make it even oilier or that will clog your pores. When you clean your skin, you want to remove oils, not replace them. You also want to make sure that you avoid comedegenic ingredients.

What Cleansing Products Are the Big Cosmetics Companies Selling for Oily Skin? One of the best things that has happened in the cosmetics industry in recent years is a genuine awareness that cleansing creams are totally inappropriate for oily skin. Until recently, if a woman with oily skin went out to buy a cleanser, there was no guarantee that she wasn't going to be sent home with an emollient-laden cream. A fair number of cases of cosmetic acne later, this is much less likely to happen now.

Cream cleansers are totally off limits for oily skin, even for removing makeup. If you have very oily skin, you shouldn't be applying heavy oil-based foundation makeup anyway. And because makeup formulated for oily skin is mostly water-based, there should be no need of a cream cleanser.

The new cleansing products formulated for oily skin and sold at cosmetics counters are sometimes called gels or foams. They are usually labeled "Rinse Off" and are promoted as being able to remove makeup as well as surface oils.

If you visit a cosmetics counter, typically you will be told that you have to fight against clogged pores and that plain old soap and water doesn't do the job because it doesn't get down deep enough into the pores. You may also be told, as I was, that soap and water can activate the sebaceous glands. These are some of the reasons that might be given for using these new "oily" skin cleansers.

Some of these "oily" cleansing products sold by the big names in skin care are probably very effective cleansers. But they are also very expensive, and like their less expensive drugstore cleansers, they are for the most part formulated from detergent-type ingredients. I can see no advantage to using them, particularly because so many of the drugstore cleansing products are recommended by dermatologists and have been used successfully for many years.

It's important for the woman with oily skin to recognize that only those products that contain over-the-counter drug ingredients, proven to be effective against acne, can make an anti-acne claim. Therefore, if an expensive department store cleansing product says it can control acne, it must contain an anti-acne ingredient such as benzoyl peroxide, salicylic acid, or resorcinol. Consumers should realize that there is a great variety of over-the-counter anti-acne drug products sold in drugstores that are significantly less expensive.

Your Oily Skin Care Routine

How Often to Cleanse Your Face If your skin is mildly to moderately oily, you will need to wash your face at least twice a day. But if your skin is oilier than that, it is often advisable to also use a toner or astringent during the day to wipe away excess oils.

Before Going to Bed
   Step 1. Using lukewarm water, splash your face at least five times to soften the top layer of your skin.
   Step 2. Using your cleansing product, with your fingertips or a soft washcloth, work up a lather on your face. Use gentle circular motions and do it as quickly as possible; it shouldn't take more than fifteen to twenty seconds. Splash your face to remove soap and wipe off the excess with a wet washcloth.
   Step 3. Splash your face with lukewarm water another fifteen times.
   Step 4. Pat your face dry with a soft towel.
   Step 5. Moisten a clean cottonball with your favorite toner and gently wipe it over your face, paying particular attention to your oily areas.
   Do not use a moisturizer or a night cream.
   Women with moderately or mildly oily skin can use a noncomedegenic product on the dry spots around the eyes. The best bet is still petrolatum. Another choice is Ar-Ex eye cream, which is a petrolatum-based product.
   If this regimen dries out your skin too much, eliminate the toner. If your skin still feels so dry that you feel you need a moisturizer, then you probably have normal, and not oily, skin.

When You Wake Up Repeat Steps 1–5 as for the night.

Step 6. Apply a noncomedegenic sunscreen with an appropriate SPF whenever you are exposed to ultraviolet light.

If you want to use makeup, apply only a water-based foundation and/or absorbent powder on your face. Make certain that all your makeup products are noncomedegenic.

Midday or Late Afternoon for Those with Very Oily Skin Moisten a clean cottonball with your favorite toner or astringent and wipe it over the oily areas of your face. If necessary, reapply foundation and/or powder.

Twice a week: Use a scrub product, following instructions on pages 216–17.

Once a week if necessary: Use an oil-absorbing clay mask, following instructions on page 218.

Choosing Your Basic Cleansing Product

In my opinion, if you have oily skin, your basic cleansing product should be a soap or detergent-type cleanser that has little or no added emolliency.

Exactly which cleansing product you choose should be determined by how oily your skin is.

Cleansing Products for Acne Women with oily skin who have acne can best be advised by a dermatologist. If you have mild acne, it can sometimes be controlled by using nothing more complicated than a benzoyl peroxide soap. Either your dermatologist or your druggist can be very helpful in suggesting appropriate products. Remember, that if you are using an over-the-counter acne medication such as benzoyl peroxide, you shouldn't be combining it with other anti-acne ingredients that might be included in a medicated bar without the guidance of your dermatologist, who might suggest a nonmedicated cleanser such as Cetaphil.

Cleansing Products for Very Oily Skin

Cetaphil—This is a relatively mild lipid-free cleansing product and is often recommended by dermatologists for very oily or acne-prone skin when used in combination with a drying product such as benzoyl peroxide.

Fostex Medicated Cleansing Bar—This contains 2 percent sulfur, 2 percent salicylic acid, boric acid, docusate sodium, and urea. This is a nonbenzoyl-peroxide medicated bar.

Aveeno Medicated Cleansing Bar—This soap-free bar contains 2 percent sulfur, 2 percent salicylic acid, and 50 percent colloidal oatmeal.

Cleansing Products for Moderately Oily Skin

Aveeno Cleansing Bar (oily skin formula)—This nonmedicated cleansing bar contains oatmeal.

Neutrogena for Oily Skin

pHisoderm Liquid (oily skin formula)—This is a soap-free pH-adjusted cleansing product.

Cleansing Products for Normal-to-Oily Skin

Cetaphil

pHisoderm Liquid (regular formula)

Purpose

Oily Skin and Astringents or Toning Lotions—Do You Need One?

Absolutely. Because they are so efficient in wiping away surface oil, toners are very useful for women with oily skin. There are, however, some things the consumer should be aware of.

Many, if not all toners, contain coal tar dyes. These colors can be comedegenic and/or irritating.

Some toners contain ingredients such as camphor, menthol, sodium borate, etc. All of these are potentially irritating and have no proven effect on the course of pimples or acne breakouts.

Although a toner, or astringent, will wipe away superficial oils, it will not by itself change the course of an acne breakout unless it contains an approved anti-acne drug.

Some toners do contain over-the-counter anti-acne drugs, such as salicylic acid used alone or in combination with sulfur or resorcinol. Salicylic acid, which is allowed in concentrations of 0.5 to 2 percent, does seem to have an anti-inflammatory effect on pimples and would appear to help speed up clearing. However, if you have acne, you should not mix and match your anti-acne ingredients. In other words, don't use a benzoyl peroxide soap with a salicylic acid astringent unless your dermatologist advises it.

Some Toners and Astringents for Oily Skin

Almay (different strengths for different degrees of oiliness)

Clearasil Medicated Astringent (medicated formula containing salicylic acid)

Estée Lauder In-Control T-Zone Solution

Lancôme Contrôle Regulating Liquid (very oily)

Lancôme Tonique Fraîcheur (mildy oily)

Some Alcohol-Free Toners for Mildly Oily Skin

Adrien Arpel Lemon and Lime Freshener

Clarins Toning Lotion for Oily/Combination Skin

Using a Scrub If You Have Oily Skin

If controlling oiliness and keeping pores unclogged is a priority for your skin, then scrubs can be very effective. The only problem is that many women tend to treat their faces as though they were inanimate objects, and they scrub too hard and too long. Scrubs are great, but only when they are used carefully, without irritating the skin. Even the oiliest skin shouldn't be subjected to a scrub more than two or three times a week, and then for no more than thirty or forty seconds of gentle rubbing.

Some products marketed for oily skin are too abrasive. If the product hurts, it may be harming your skin. On the other hand, if a scrub contains too many creams, it can be too greasy for oily skin. That's why I like best the old-fashioned scrubs with no additional ingredients.

Some Scrubs for Oily Skin

oatmeal (great for polishing the skin)

Adrien Arpel Sea Kelp Cleanser

Buf-Puf

Clinique Exfoliating Scrub

Acne and Scrubs

Rubbing at acne-prone skin can irritate existing comedones and induce new ones. If you have acne, the safest path you can follow is to forgo scrubs unless your dermatologist advises otherwise. Many dermatologists feel that acne skin is very easily abraded and damaged and specifically advise against abrasive scrubs. In one study, five abrasive products were tested over a period of eight weeks. At the end of that time, it was found that "none of the test materials had a clinically significant effect in eliminating comedones." It is interesting to note that at the beginning of the study, all the ingredients had the effect of reducing comedones to some extent. Unfortunately, in some of these patients, this reduction was followed by an increase in inflamed comedones.

Masks for Oily Skin

Rinse-Off Masks   Clay and fuller's-earth-type masks certainly do absorb oils and make the skin glow. Cleansing masks are fun, and one of the nice things about having oily skin is being able to use them to remove old skin cells. All these drying clay masks are made of essentially the same type of ingredients, and I can see little justification in indulging in the higher-priced items.

Some Rinse-Off Masks

Adrien Arpel Sea Mud Masque

Mudd Mask

Shiseido Mask

Peel-Off Masks   Some experts believe that peel-off masks stretch and pull the skin and therefore are not advisable, even for oily skin. However, many women love them because something about exfoliating and pulling off all those dead skin cells is very gratifying. They are not necessary for good skin care.

Cleansing Guidelines for Normal Skin

The first rule of caring for normal skin is: Don't upset the balance. Keep your cleansing products simple, and don't use anything that is very drying or anything that is overwhelmingly comedegenic. And, most important, don't tempt the fates by indulging in any overkill skin care routines, including the excessive use of cleansers, masks, or scrubs.

Cream Cleansers I think I made it clear that I am not a fan of cream cleansers for any skin type. However, if you wear a lot of makeup and feel that you want to use a cream cleanser, at least some of the time, take a look at the list of products on page 209.

Your Normal Skin Care Routine

Before Going to Bed

Step 1. Using lukewarm water, splash your face at least five times to soften the top layer of your skin.

Step 2. Using your cleansing product, with your fingertips or a soft washcloth, work up a lather on your face. Use gentle circular motions and do it as quickly as possible; it shouldn't take more than fifteen to twenty seconds. Splash your face to remove soap and wipe off the excess with a wet washcloth.

Step 3. Splash your face with lukewarm water another fifteen times.

Step 4. Remove excess water by patting with a soft towel, but don't dry thoroughly.

Step 5. Apply a light moisturizer over your entire face. If you want, you can also use an eye cream such as Ar-Ex or vaseline in the eye area.

When You Wake Up Repeat Steps 1–5 as in the evening.

Step 6. Apply a light moisturizer over your entire face before applying makeup.

Step 7. Apply a sunscreen with an appropriate SPF whenever you are exposed to ultraviolet light.

Once a week: Use a scrub product as suggested on the next page.

Choosing Your Basic Cleansing Product

If you have normal skin, you want to steer away from both extremes in soap products—drying soaps designed for oily skin and heavily emollient soaps better suited to dry skin. Here are some mild middle-of-the-road choices.

Cetaphil

Dove

Lowila

Neutrogena (regular)

pHisoderm (regular)

Purpose

Using a Scrub on Normal Skin

Yes, you definitely should use a scrub to exfoliate dead skin cells, improve circulation, and bring a polish to your skin. But what may start out as a simple way of putting a glow to your cheeks all too often becomes a highly energetic and intense exercise that may do your skin more harm than good. The word is *caution!* A woman with normal skin should use a scrub no more than twice a week and the technique should be limited to under thirty seconds for the *entire* face.

Scrubs for Normal Skin

cornmeal

oatmeal (This is still wonderful as far as I'm concerned. If your skin dries out too much for oatmeal, you can thin it with a small amount of moisturizer.)

Adrien Arpel Honey and Almond Scrub

Buf-Puf (gentle or regular, depending upon skin sensitivity)

Cleansing Masks for Normal Skin

If you have normal skin, a cleansing mask isn't an essential part of your cleansing routine and it may be too drying for all but your T-zone. However, women enjoy using masks perhaps because they imply a certain amount of glamour—we've all seen photographs of sophisticated women at expensive spas with globs of green goo on their faces. Should you decide to use a cleansing mask, don't do it too often—no more than once every couple of weeks—don't keep it on too long, and stay away from products that are exceptionally drying. Women with skin that is in the normal-to-dry range should always be careful to rinse off all the mask and immediately apply a moisturizer. And if you have pores that really need a clay mask, you may have combination or mildly oily skin and should be treating it accordingly.

Some Rinse-Off Cleansing Masks for Normal Skin

Payot Clay Clarifying Clay Mask

Shiseido Facial Masque

Toners for Normal Skin

A woman with normal skin rarely needs a toner, and when she does it is primarily in her T-zone. You may also need a toner to help remove cleansing creams, if you insist upon using them, and during the summer if your skin becomes more oily. Most of the time you can get away with a less strong toner, even on your T-zone, and your cheeks may rarely if ever need to be toned.

Some Toners for Normal Skin

witch hazel

Clarins Toning Lotion for Normal Skin

Lancôme Tonique Fraîcheur (alcohol-based)

Lancôme Tonique Douceur (nonalcohol)

Cleansing Guidelines for Combination-Type Skin

If you have combination-type skin, and most of us do, then you have to understand both dry and oily skin. Read the sections directed at oily and dry skin. Look at your skin and decide, how oily is the oily part? How dry is the dry? These are the questions that the woman with combination skin has to answer for herself before choosing cleansing products. If you are one of those rare women with an exceptionally oily T-zone and exceptionally dry skin around the side of the face, then you may literally have to use two separate sets of products. Fortunately, combination skin is usually not that extreme.

Your goal with combination skin is to keep the T-zone free of oils and free of pimples and clogged pores without drying out the rest of your face.

Your Combination Skin Care Routine

Before You Go to Bed

Step 1. Using lukewarm water, splash your face at least five times to soften the top layer of your skin.

Step 2. Using your cleansing product, with your fingertips or a soft washcloth, work up a lather on your face. Use gentle circular motions and do it as quickly as possible; it shouldn't take more than fifteen to twenty seconds. Splash your face to remove soap and wipe off the excess moisture with a wet washcloth.

Step 3. Splash your face with lukewarm water another fifteen times.

Step 4. Pat your face dry with a soft towel.

Step 5. Use a light, noncomedegenic moisturizer *only* on those parts of your face where the skin is dry.

Step 6. Moisten a clean cottonball with your favorite toner or astringent and wipe it over the oily areas of your face. If you want, you can use a noncomedegenic eye cream such as petrolatum or Ar-Ex Eye Cream.

When You Wake Up Repeat Steps 1–6 as you did at night.
Step 7. Apply a noncomedegenic sunscreen with an appropriate SPF whenever you are exposed to ultraviolet light.

What kind of makeup a woman with combination skin can use depends on how oily her T-zone is. Someone with a very oily T-zone should stick to powder or a water-based foundation. Remember to use only non-comedegenic products on your oily areas.

Twice a week: Use a scrub product as needed.
Once a week: A deep-cleaning clay mask can be used on your T-zone. Allow at least a day to elapse between using a scrub and a mask.

Choosing Your Major Cleansing Product

Before deciding on your particular cleansing product, you have to determine whether your skin is best described as mildly oily T-zone and normal-to-dry elsewhere or very oily T-zone and normal-to-oily elsewhere.

Some Cleansers for Mildly Oily T-zone and Dry-to-Normal Skin Elsewhere

Cetaphil

Neutrogena (regular)

Purpose

Some Cleansers for Very Oily T-zone and Normal-to-Oily Skin Elsewhere

Cetaphil

Neutrogena (oily-skin formula)

Combination-Type Skin and Astringents and Toning Lotions—Do You Need One?

Toning lotions are extremely useful for the woman with combination skin. Not only do they help keep the T-zone clear of her skin's natural oils, but they can also be used to wipe away moisturizers and other oily products that might be applied to the non-T-zone area. What kind of toning lotion to use is determined by how clogged the pores get. If you have a very oily T-zone, read the suggestions for oily skin on page 215.

Toning Lotions for Moderately Oily T-zones

Almay

Dior Hydro Dior Lotion Stimulante

Estée Lauder In-Control T-zone solution

Lancôme Tonique Fraîcheur

Toning Lotions for Mildly Oily T-zones

witch hazel

Adrien Arpel Lemon and Lime Freshener

Clarins Toning Lotion for Oily/Combination Skin

Using a Scrub on Combination-Type Skin

Here are some suggestions:

ground cornmeal

oatmeal

Adrien Arpel Sea Kelp Cleanser

Buf-Puf (regular or gentle, depending on your skin)

Masks for Combination-Type Skin

Rinse-off masks are wonderful for combination-type skin, but if your non-T-zone is dry-to-normal, use rinse-off cleansing masks in your T-zone only.

Some Cleansing Masks for Oily T-zones

Adrien Arpel Sea Mud Pack

Mudd Mask

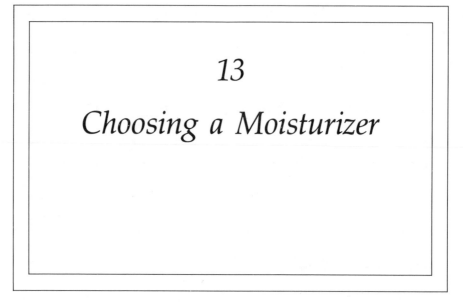

13

Choosing a Moisturizer

Let Your Skin Type, and Your Pocketbook, Be Your Guides

When you go out to buy a moisturizer, there are two basic considerations.

1. What is your skin type?

Skin care ads that typically show a young woman with flawless skin holding up the latest anti-aging product are very misleading. The message seems to be that everyone, even a young woman, with nary a dry spot, let alone a wrinkle, needs to use these heavy-duty moisturizing products. This is simply not true.

Moisturizers are meant to relieve dry skin. They are not designed for women with oily skin; they have natural oils protecting their skin. Nor are they for women with normal-to-oily skin. The fact is that most young women under twenty-five have normal-to-oily skin. And if you have oily, acne-prone skin, no matter what your age, you want to stay away from most of the ingredients that are included in the typical moisturizing product. On the other hand, if you are over forty and you have dry, mature skin, you want to buy and use a protective moisturizing cream.

Women with normal-to-dry skin will probably be happiest with a moisturizing lotion. Women over twenty five with normal-to-oily skin will want to choose a lotion that is specifically noncomedegenic.

2. How much do you want to spend?

Twelve ounces of Nivea Moisturizing Lotion will cost you less than $4. One ounce of La Prairie's Cellular Day Cream will cost you approximately $70. Money is very much a factor in deciding which moisturizer to buy.

Many dermatologists feel that petrolatum is the best moisturizer available, and today there are many moisturizing creams and lotions that include petrolatum in formulations that are not greasy. Many of these petrolatum-based products are very reasonably priced. And they are excellent moisturizing products.

By and large, medical experts say that there is no reason to believe that the higher-priced moisturizers do a more effective job of protecting your skin. Yet women repeatedly talk about how much better their skin looks with certain moisturizers. The fact is that although the lower-priced petrolatum-based products are probably every bit as effective as, and in some instances superior to, the expensive department store moisturizers, they don't always leave your skin with the same kind of sheen or finish. Often this finish is the result of additional ingredients that add a temporary glow or reflect light in such a way that your skin looks dewier. Sometimes these expensive products do seem to enable your skin to retain moisture for a longer period of time. Sometimes it is just the way the more expensive moisturizer feels or smells that makes it particularly appealing to a consumer.

After all, books and articles on skin care have been telling the consumer that she doesn't have to spend a lot of money for moisturizers. Yet consumers continue to return to department stores and purchase high-priced creams and moisturizers. Some of this is the direct result of high-pressure sales techniques and advertising, but some of it is because steady skin care consumers like the way the products look or feel. All this means is that if you are solely interested in taking care of your skin, you can absolutely get satisfaction and superb skin protection with many of the more inexpensive products, but if you have other considerations, then you may think it worth your while to spend more.

My own solution has been to compromise—to use inexpensive petrolatum-based moisturizers for most of my skin care needs and to save the more expensive products for those times when I want a little more sheen to my skin.

When and Where to Apply Your Moisturizer

Women are sometimes confused about when and where to apply their moisturizing agent. Here are some guidelines:

Dry, mature skin—over your entire face and neck, immediately after rinsing your face, every time you wash or rinse your face, as well as before going to bed. And if it is at all feasible, at four- to five-hour intervals during the day, particularly if your face feels dry.

Dry skin—over your entire face and neck, immediately after rinsing your face, every time you wash or rinse your face, as well as before going to bed. And, if it is at all feasible, at midday, as well as any other time your face feels dry.

Normal skin—over your entire face and neck, immediately after rinsing your face, every time you wash or rinse your face, as well as before going to bed and any other time your face feels dry.

Combination skin—*only* over those parts of your face and neck that are dry whenever you wash or rinse your face. Never apply a moisturizer to the parts of your face that are oily.

Oily skin—Guess what, you shouldn't use a moisturizer. Oily skin is oily skin, and you have no need of more oils.

Oily acne skin—Oily, acne-prone skin certainly doesn't need a moisturizer. However, there is an exception to this rule. While some women are undergoing acne treatment with drying ingredients such as benzoyl peroxide, the skin becomes so dry that it needs a moisturizer, in which case it should be applied as directed by your dermatologist in those areas that have become exceptionally dry.

If You Have Dry Skin

Women with dry skin need a moisturizer with a good occlusive agent such as petrolatum or lanolin. These ingredients will reduce evaporation from the skin.

One of the first things to decide is whether you want a lotion or a cream. Creams are thicker and richer than lotions, which, of course, have more water. Several companies make almost identical products in both a cream and a lotion.

If your skin is very dry and mature, you will probably be happier with a cream. But there are other times when a woman with normal-to-dry skin might prefer a cream over a lotion. For instance, a cream offers more protection in the winter, particularly if one is going to be outdoors. It is also a good choice in dry climates as well as in airplanes or offices with dry heat.

A woman with moderately or mildly dry skin will probably prefer a lotion because it is lighter.

If you have dry skin and are friendly with your pharmacist, ask them to make a mixture, which is inexpensive, of hydrophilic ointment and water.

Creams and Oils—Drugstore

Allercreme Ultra-Emollient Cream (mineral oil, petrolatum, lanolin)

Cutemol Cream (liquid petrolatum, acetylated lanolin, isopropyl myristate)

Nivea Skin Oil (mineral oil, petrolatum, lanolin)

Purpose Dry Skin Cream (mineral oil, petrolatum, almond oil)

Lotions—Drugstore

Lubriderm (water, mineral oil, petrolatum)

Sofenol 5 (mineral oil, petrolatum, glycerin)

Wondra Lotion (petrolatum, lanolin acid, glycerin)

Moisturizers—Department Store

Clarins Cell Extracts Moisturizing Cream

Lancôme Hydrix (petrolatum, mineral oil, hydrogenated lanolin)

La Prairie Day Cream

If You Have Normal Skin

If you have normal skin, you probably want a lotion, rather than a cream. You should also choose a product that is lighter. Here are some choices:

Moisturizing Lotions—Drugstore

Complex 15 (mineral oil, glycerin, glyceryl stearate, lecithin)

Keri Light (glycerin, stearyl alcohol/ceteareth 20)

Moisturel (petrolatum, glycerin)

Moisturizers—Department Store

Clarins Cell Extracts Moisturizing Base (lotion)

Clinique Dramatically Different

Lancôme's Progrès Plus

La Prairie Skin Conditioner

If You Have Combination-Type Skin

First of all, you want to be careful not to apply your moisturizer in your T-zone. Ideally, you should choose a moisturizer that is not laden with comedegenic ingredients because you don't want to risk having it slide over to your T-zone and cause pimples.

If your non-T-zone is really dry, choose a moisturizer from the list intended for normal or dry skin.

Moisturizers—Drugstore

Moisturel (petrolatum, glycerin, dimethicone)

Neutrogena Moisturizer

Sea Breeze Moisture Lotion "99% oil free" (glycerin, aloe vera gel)

Wibi (glycerin, SD alcohol 40)

Moisturizers—Department Store

Adrien Arpel Oil Blotting Lotion

Clinique Skin Texture Lotion

Lancôme Bienfait du Matin (for normal or oily skin)

If You Have Oily Skin

Most of the time, you don't need to use a moisturizer, except possibly around your eyes. There are, however, some exceptions to this.

If You Are Undergoing Acne Treatment That Dries Your Skin

Some women who are undergoing benzoyl peroxide therapy for acne complain that their skin becomes too dry. If that happens, your dermatologist may have a product to recommend. Dr. James Fulton, who runs the Face Up Centers, specializing in the treatment of acne, markets a moisturizer he recommends for just such a purpose. It's a light, petrolatum-based product. You can get a brochure and order products by calling 1-800-222-SKIN. If you live in California, the number is 1-800-221-SKIN. Neutrogena has recently marketed a product designed for women undergoing acne therapy; it can be found in most drugstores. Moisturel, a non-comedegenic petrolatum-based product, is another possibility.

What About the New Noncomedegenic Moisturizing and Anti-Aging Products for Oily Skin?

There is a whole new category of skin care product—noncomedegenic "moisturizers" for oily skin that are alcohol-based. These products are geared to helping reduce oils. Some of them may also include some of the "hot" new ingredients such as vitamin A or collagen or cholesterol.

Some of these include too many drying ingredients such as alcohol to be considered true moisturizers, and I don't think they should be considered as such. Perhaps the product receiving the most attention right now is Estée Lauder's Equalizer Oil-Free HydroGel. The ingredients include water, alcohol, propylene glycol, and mixed phospholipids. Other ingredients include retinyl palmitate (vitamin A palmitate).

Revlon's Moon Drops also has an anti-aging product for oily skin. This product contains a sunscreen, but it does not have an SPF number, and one assumes that the concentration is not sufficient for the product to be used as a sunscreen. It contains a great number of ingredients, including propylene glycol, alcohol, and vitamin E.

If you read the ingredients of these or most of the other products formulated for oily skin, you will see that they rarely include an occlusive such as mineral oil or petrolatum and instead rely upon humectants for moisturizing.

What About Moisturizers That Include Sunscreens?

Certain department store moisturizers, particularly those that say they help prevent premature aging caused by environmental factors, such as the sun, contain sunscreens. Many of them do not contain sunscreen ingredients in adequate concentrations to qualify as FDA-approved sunscreen products. In order to be a bona fide sunscreen, the product must be classified as an over-the-counter drug. Such a sunscreen will be labeled accordingly and will have an SPF number on the labeling.

There seems to be a push in the direction of combining the two functions of sunscreen and moisturizer in one product, and several manufacturers are attempting to do that. Elizabeth Arden, for example, has launched Immunage, a moisturizer with a sunscreen with SPF 15.

I think these bona fide moisturizer-type sunscreens are very valid and useful when a woman is going to be outdoors. Whether you need an SPF number 15 in a moisturizer to be worn around the home or office is another matter, and one the consumer should consider before choosing these products.

What About Moisturizing Masks?

There are several companies that manufacture products described as "moisturizing masks" or "pick-up masks." To be honest, I don't like to advise women to use these products for several reasons. They are obviously the wrong choice for skin that is oily or on the oily side. For women with dry skin, some of these are peel-offs, and I don't think all that stretching and pulling is good for the skin. I honestly prefer the plain old-fashioned moisturizing masks that you just apply to the skin because you want a facial. The commercial masks frequently have a real mishmash of ingredients, and I don't believe in using anything more than necessary. In my experience, I have found that women buy these products, use them once or twice, and then forget about them. Sometimes they make the skin itch or tingle. Other times, the effects are so temporary or elusive that it hardly seems worth the bother. I love homemade moisturizing masks because I believe they are more reliable and less likely to irritate the skin.

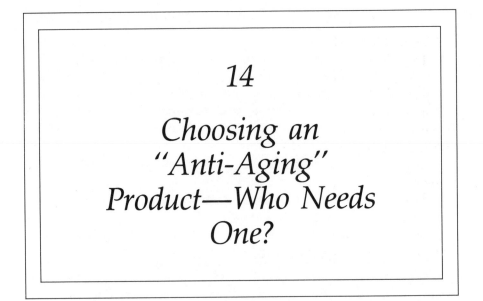

14

Choosing an "Anti-Aging" Product—Who Needs One?

Everyone, according to some skin care companies. No one, according to some critics of the skin care industry. My own point of view? If you are under thirty or have oily or acne-prone skin, then you don't need to purchase one of these so-called super creams. However, if you are over thirty, and you don't have oily, acne-prone skin and don't break out from the product, and can afford to experiment with skin care products, there is probably no harm, and there might be some good.

Which one to use? This is a matter for you and your pocketbook to decide. One of these products may make your skin look better, but remember, even the skin care companies indicate that this effect is temporary and will disappear once you stop using the product.

If you're in the market for expensive skin care products, the following list includes some of the most well known. Most of the products in this list were "cited" by the FDA as having gone over the line in terms of products claims.

These are also some of the more expensive skin care products currently marketed. Some of the "important" ingredients are listed with each product so that you can more easily decide which one you might want to use.

· Avon's BioAdvance Beauty Recovery System
    Ingredients include: retinol, beta carotene, retinyl acetate, retinyl palmitate.

- Christian Dior's Capture
  Ingredients include: thymus extracts, collagen and elastin peptides, "packaged"-in liposomes.
- Avon's Collagen Booster Line Controlling Lotion
  Ingredients include: ascorbic acid, hydroxypropyocellulose, panthenol.
- Shiseido's B.H.–24 (Day/Night)
  Ingredients include: hyaluronic acid, sunscreen (day).
- Biotherm's Energie Active Age Protector
  Ingredients include: tocopherol (vitamin E), UVA and UVB sunscreens.
- Clarins's Double Serum Multi-Regenerant
  Ingredients include: vegetable oils, bovine spleen extract, panthenol.
- Estée Lauder's Eyezone Repair Gel
  Ingredients include: "Tissue Matrix Fluid," vitamin A palmitate.
- Estée Lauder's Future Perfect
  Ingredients include: sodium hyaluronate (hyaluronic acid), retinyl palmitate (vitamin A), tocopherol linoleate (vitamin E), "Lift Serum/Anti-Wrinkle Complex."
- Chanel's Lift Serum
  Ingredients include: plastoderm, "a complex which incorporates a balance of natural proteins and carbohydrates."
- Prescriptives's Line Preventor
  Ingredients include: vitamin A, vitamin E, sodium hyaluronate.
- Lancôme's Niosôme Système Anti-Age
  Ingredients include: niosomes.
- Discipline's Pro-Cell T
  Ingredients include: thymus extracts, vitamins, collagen, elastin.
- La Prairie's Skin Caviar
  Ingredients include: vitamins A and E, panthenol pro-vitamin B-5.

A Moisturizer and an Anti-Aging Product

Companies sometimes recommend using moisturizers along with their anti-aging products, and the promotional literature will suggest applying a moisturizer after the anti-aging cream. I've spoken to a good number of women over forty or fifty, with dry skin, who did and who discovered that you are never too old to get pimples. Sometimes the combination can be too "rich" for even very dry skin. I personally do not combine a moisturizer and an anti-aging product. I use the super cream before bedtime, and moisturizers during the day.

Remember, that all of these creams are cosmetics, and they cannot promise anything more than temporary results. There is, however, a new drug product that promises more.

Retin-A—The Pros and the Cons

In the world of wrinkles, 1988 will go down in history as the year of Retin-A, the prescription drug manufactured by Johnson & Johnson. In January of that year, a report was published in the prestigious *Journal of the American Medical Association* that suggested that dermatological researchers had found a cure for the common wrinkle. Researchers at the University of Michigan reported that a study showed dramatic results from treating sun-damaged skin with Retin-A. Thirty men and women, aged thirty-five to seventy, were used in this study. Half of them applied Retin-A to their faces once a day; the other half used a similar cream, but without the drug. After several months, the group using Retin-A showed significant skin changes, including noticeably fewer wrinkles.

For the first time, something was available to reverse the effects of photoaging, and all across America, women, and men, responded by lining up at dermatologists' offices in an attempt to turn back the hands of time. Sales went through the ceiling as pharmacists began reporting shortages of the drug.

Until 1988, Retin-A, a vitamin A derivative, was best known as an effective anti-acne drug, typically prescribed for teenagers with skin problems. The person most responsible for developing Retin-A is Dr. Albert M. Kligman, the noted University of Pennsylvania dermatologist who is often called the dean of dermatology. Kligman began using Retin-A as an acne medication almost twenty years ago, and reports from his patients are what prompted him to begin to use the drug on sun-damaged skin.

The Pros

According to its advocates, Retin-A accelerates cell turnover, stimulates blood vessel growth, and boosts production of collagen and elastin. The end result is a general tightening of the skin as well as fewer wrinkles. Retin-A would appear to be effective also against brown spots and other forms of photoaging. And there is some promising research taking place to study the effects of Retin-A against actinic keratoses, a form of skin cancer caused by the sun.

At this time, Retin-A is FDA-approved only for the treatment of acne, although tests are now being conducted to determine whether it has additional uses.

The Cons

Although most dermatologists are enthusiastic about the results that they have obtained from use of Retin-A, a few are less convinced that Retin-A is all that effective. Many patients who used Retin-A have complained that it made their skin excessively dry and red-looking, particularly at the beginning of the treatment, and, in the study group, a few people experienced results distressing enough to make them drop out. Others required topical anti-inflammatories. Patients have complained of stinging as well as a burning feeling in the eyes. Some dermatologists have begun to reduce concentrations and mix Retin-A with moisturizers to lessen chapping and irritation. However, some feel that unless the skin is allowed to react and peel, the benefits will be minimal.

If you stop using Retin-A, your skin will gradually go back to its previous condition.

Once you begin using Retin-A, you have to accept the fact that Retin-A thins the outermost layers of the epidermis, allowing more penetration of ultraviolet light. Making a commitment to Retin-A means that you must commit yourself to never again going in the sun without a sunscreen with an SPF of at least 15.

Retin-A peels off the outermost layer of the skin, and for darker-skinned women this can mean a change in color of their skin.

If you go on a regimen of Retin-A, expect to become much more involved with your dermatologist, whom you will typically visit every few months to monitor your treatment.

Caution: To date, there have been no well-controlled studies of the effects of Retin-A on pregnant women. If you are pregnant or planning to become pregnant, it may not be advisable to use this drug until it has been proven safe and effective. Retin-A is in the same family of drugs as Accutane (see page 253). Studies performed on rats and rabbits who were given doses significantly higher than the human dose have revealed no evidence of impaired fertility or fetal harm. According to *Drug Facts and Comparisons,* 1988 ed., there was, however, "a slightly higher incidence of irregularly contoured or partially ossified skull bones in some fetuses."

How Retin-A Is Typically Prescribed

Most dermatologists say that it takes from three to six months before one can see the full effects of Retin-A, and they often caution their patients that the Retin-A treatment will probably be lifelong. Many dermatologists start out by telling their patients to use Retin-A on their skin every other night. After about four to six weeks, they may up this to every night. During the day, the patient is usually told to use a moisturizer to counteract the drying effect of the medication. After a year, use of Retin-A is often cut back to a maintenance level, which can vary from two to four times a week.

Patients using Retin-A are told always to use a number 15 sunscreen and are cautioned against using other types of cosmetic products that might be drying, such as astringents, toners, abrasives, and harsh cleansers.

Some other cautions for someone using Retin-A:

·   Consult your dermatologist before attempting any methods of facial hair removal, including wax, cream depilatories, or electrolysis.
·   Remember that Retin-A-treated skin is more likely to be sensitive to climates that are dry, hot, or cold.
·   Consult your dermatologist about appropriate cosmetic products, including cleansers and moisturizers. Some dermatologists feel that their Retin-A patients have a greater tendency to become sensitive to the ingredients in skin care products.
·   Cleanse gently and avoid harsh fabrics and washcloths.
·   Consult with your dermatologist before bleaching, dyeing, or perming your hair; if you get a medical go-ahead, warn your beautician to take special care to avoid getting chemicals on Retin-A-treated skin.
·   Call your dermatologist if you experience redness, stinging, or irritation.
·   Don't borrow someone else's Retin-A, and don't allow anyone to use your prescription.

What Is Retin-A? What Is Not?

Because Retin-A is in the same family as vitamin A, some consumers have become confused in distinguishing between the two. Vitamin A has been included in cosmetic products for a good number of years as retinyl, retinyl acetate, or retinyl palmitate. These ingredients are not drugs and do not have the same effects as Retin-A.

Retin-A is available by prescription only. Therefore, at least for the time being, you're not going to find it in any cosmetic skin care product.

Products that currently include retinol (vitamin A) or another form of vitamin A are: Estée Lauder's Eyezone Repair Gel and Future Perfect; Prescriptives's Flight Cream and Skin Renewal Cream; Avon's BioAdvance; and Lancaster's Suractif cream, as well as a good number of vitamin A and D creams sold at drugstores. On a recent trip through a drugstore, I noticed several creams that used phrases such as retinyl therapy. Remember, Retin-A is available by prescription only. The language on these creams can be very misleading to someone who hasn't been informed about the difference.

15

If You Have Acne

Every teenager in America is probably familiar with over-the-counter acne preparations, but often adult women resist the word acne and are not familiar with these medications. Because they have been tested and received drug status, they are considered safe and effective for acne treatment.

If you have moderate to severe acne, you should see a dermatologist for diagnosis and guidance, but if you have mild acne that primarily consists of closed comedones, you may decide that the first thing you want to do is to try some of the over-the-counter preparations. Fortunately, there are over-the-counter medications that have been shown to be safe and effective for the treatment of acne and have been placed in the category of over-the-counter drug. As drugs, they had to be classified as safe and effective in order to make an anti-acne claim. In order to do this, an advisory review panel was formed, reporting to the FDA, and charged with determining which ingredients marketed for acne conditions could be termed safe and effective.

For use as over-the-counter acne medication, the panel has, to date, reviewed about twenty-seven ingredients included in a wide range of products that were submitted to the FDA to receive over-the-counter drug status. These ingredients, as are other ingredients submitted for drug status, were classified in one of the three following ways:

Category I: Generally recognized as safe and effective for the claimed therapeutic indication.

Category II: Not generally recognized as safe and effective or making unacceptable claims.

Category III: Insufficient data available to permit final classification.

The following list of ingredients are the ones that the FDA has named as safe and effective in over-the-counter acne products:

benzoyl peroxide 2.5 to 10 percent

resorcinol 2 percent in certain combinations

resorcinol monacetate 3 percent in certain combinations

salicylic acid 0.5 to 2 percent

sulfur 3 to 10 percent

sulfur 3 to 8 percent in certain combinations

All of these ingredients exfoliate the skin and induce peeling. They are obviously very drying. They should not be used in combination because the effect may increase dryness and irritation.

Benzoyl Peroxide—The Most Popular Over-the-Counter Drug for Acne

Benzoyl peroxide, which is considered safe and effective in the appropriate strengths, is one of the simplest and most effective methods now available for the treatment of acne. As a matter of fact, for many cases of acne, I'm told that it is sometimes all that is necessary.

Benzoyl peroxide affects acne skin in two ways: Because it is a peroxide, it releases oxygen, some of which reaches down into the sebaceous follicle and delivers a deadly punch to those anaerobic bacteria that are lurking there. And benzoyl peroxide is an exfoliant, causing peeling of the stratum corneum.

Numerous studies have been done to evaluate the effects of benzoyl peroxide, and the consistent pattern has been improvement in the majority of patients treated. When one double-blind study of acne patients was conducted, no other form of treatment was used except washing with soap and water before one to four applications of 5.5 percent benzoyl peroxide per day (the number of applications was dependent upon the response of the individual skin, taking into consideration the amount of peeling as well as any irritation). Evaluation of this study showed that the acne of 65 percent of those treated with benzoyl peroxide improved; that of 29 percent remained the same; and that of 6 percent was worse.

In another study, patients with grade 2 and grade 3 acne (for acne ratings, see page 99) were evaluated based upon actual lesion counts as well as overall impression. In this study, patients treated with 5 percent benzoyl peroxide had a 39.7 percent improvement rate after six weeks, as opposed to a 7.7 percent improvement rate in the control group.

Further, it would appear from these studies that benzoyl peroxide is effective against all types of acne lesions.

Most dermatologists with whom I spoke recommended benzoyl peroxide as the most effective over-the-counter treatment for acne. Benzoyl peroxide comes in three strengths: 2.5 percent, 5 percent, and 10 percent. These numbers refer to the concentration of benzoyl peroxide in the product. Benzoyl peroxide is found in different forms, including cleansers, lotions, creams, and gels.

Over-the-counter benzoyl peroxide cleansers include:

Fostex 10% Wash (liquid)

Fostex 10% (cleansing bar)

Oxy 10 Wash (liquid)

PanOxyl 5% (cleansing bar)

PanOxyl 10% (cleansing bar)

Over-the-counter benzoyl peroxide lotions include:

Acne-10

Benoxyl 5

Benoxyl 10

Clearasil 10%

Dry and Clear (5%)

Loroxide (5.5%)

Oxy 5

Oxy 10

Vanoxide (5%)

Over-the-counter benzoyl peroxide creams include:

Acne-Aid (10%)

Clearasil Maximum Strength (10%)

Cuticura Acne (5%)

Dry and Clear Double Strength

Fostex (10%)

Oxy 10 Cover

Over-the-counter benzoyl peroxide gels include:

Clear by Design (2.5%)

Del Aqua-5

Del Aqua-10

Fostex 5%

Fostex 10%

Xerac BP5

Xerac BP10

Using Over-the-Counter Benzoyl Peroxide Preparations

When I was writing this chapter, I purchased a variety of benzoyl peroxide preparations and was shocked to see how few instructions came with the products. Most consumers are not clear about exactly what results they can expect.

Here's a typical question: "How do I know for certain that I'm not having an adverse reaction to benzoyl peroxide?"

Benzoyl peroxide is supposed to dry the skin, remove excess sebum, and encourage mild desquamation, but it can also cause excessive drying and peeling. Consumers are understandably uncertain about how to know the difference between an expected reaction and an adverse or allergic reaction. Here are some hints: Benzoyl peroxide may normally cause a transitory (or fleeting) feeling of warmth or stinging. It also causes dryness and some peeling. But if the skin turns excessively red, or if there is discomfort, excessive scaling, swelling, or edema, you may be having an adverse reaction and should discontinue use. I would also suggest contacting a dermatologist or calling a hospital emergency room. A physician may want to see you or it may be suggested that you can handle the discomfort with emollients such as petrolatum and cool compresses.

When using benzoyl peroxide, remember:

· Benzoyl peroxide is intended for external use only.
· Keep the product away from your eyelids, lips, mouth, or mucous membranes such as the inside of the nose.
· Do not use if your skin is inflamed without consulting a physician.
· Avoid other possible sources of skin irritation such as sunlight.
· Don't use benzoyl peroxide and another acne medication simultaneously unless directed by a physician.
· Benzoyl peroxide will stain clothing and bleach hair.
· Benzoyl peroxide can be absorbed by the skin, and should not be used by a pregnant woman or a nursing mother unless necessary and directed by a physician. Safety and efficacy in children under twelve has not been established.
· Don't use benzoyl peroxide and other cosmetics such as drying astringents and scrubs together.

Some women are sensitive to benzoyl peroxide. To determine whether you are, test the product on a small acne-affected area once a day for several days. If any excessive dryness or undue irritation develops, discontinue use until you have consulted your doctor.

Benzoyl peroxide should be used cautiously. Always start out with a small amount and gradually increase it, making sure that you are not having a reaction. *Read the label of all benzoyl peroxide products carefully. If you experience more burning or irritation than is described, discontinue use immediately and consult a physician.*

How to Use Benzoyl Peroxide Cleansers

1. Wet your face thoroughly before using the product.
2. Start by washing only once daily with a 5 percent cleanser to see how your skin tolerates the product. Do this for three or four days. (Never use benzoyl peroxide near the eyes or mucous membranes.)

3. If you are not bothered by excessive drying or peeling, wash twice a day.
4. If you want to switch to a 10 percent product, do so gradually, starting with once a day.
5. After using the cleanser, rinse thoroughly.

With benzoyl peroxide cleansers, you can control the effects by either washing less frequently or by using water to dilute the concentration.

How to Use Benzoyl Peroxide Lotions, Creams, and Gels The first thing to do, of course, is to buy the product. For beginning use, choose a product with a 5 percent concentration, or a 2.5 percent concentration, if you can find it. When using creams, lotions, or gels, keep in mind that gels are usually more drying, so you may want to begin with a cream or a lotion.

Stage One:

1. Gently wash your face with a mild nonmedicated, nonfatted soap. Do not use scrubs or abrasive products.
2. Start out with a benzoyl peroxide 5 percent product, or 2.5 percent if you can find it. Using a small amount, spread it evenly over all of the facial areas where you tend to break out. The idea is to zap not only current comedones, but also those that are beginning to form.
3. After two hours, rinse your face well to remove the benzoyl peroxide.

Do this for several days to see how well, or badly, your skin tolerates benzoyl peroxide. If there is more discomfort than is tolerable, but it is within a normal range and your skin is not excessively red, peeling, or swollen, stop using the product for a couple of days, and, when you continue use, leave it on for only one hour and use it only every other day. If you have an extreme reaction, discontinue use and consult a doctor. If there is only mild peeling and no excessive discomfort, intensify your program by moving through the following stages.

Stage Two:

1. Wash your face gently, using no abrasives, superfatted soaps, or medicated cleansers.
2. Once a day, apply a thin film of benzoyl peroxide over those areas where you are most likely to break out, avoiding the area around the eyes, the nose, and the mouth.

3. Leave it on for four hours daily.
4. Rinse off.
5. Wait five or six days to evaluate the condition of your skin. If there is no excessive peeling, redness, or discomfort, move on to Stage Three.

Stage Three:

1. Wash your face gently and apply a thin film of benzoyl peroxide as described above.
2. Leave it on for eight hours and rinse off.
3. If there is no excessive peeling, redness, or discomfort, continue doing this for several weeks.

By now, you should be seeing some results, and you may never have to increase the concentration of benzoyl peroxide or the amount of time you wear it.

If you feel that you are getting results, but you are still getting new breakouts, move up to Stage Four.

Stage Four:

1. Twice a day, wash your face gently and apply a thin film of benzoyl peroxide as described above.
2. Leave it on for six hours and rinse off.
3. Again, wait four to six weeks to evaluate the results. If you have reached maintenance level, continue for at least a month.

Keep track of all comedones, new and old. When all of your old pimples start clearing, and you are not developing any new ones, you have reached a maintenance plateau. Continue the benzoyl peroxide treatment for at least a month.

Benzoyl Peroxide and Skin Sensitivity

Occasionally, some benzoyl peroxide users discover that their skin is sensitive. Most people report a certain amount of mild burning and itching sensation, but benzoyl peroxide can produce a more acute irritation in certain women, and men, with very sensitive skin. Those with very fair skin may find themselves more sensitive; this is also true of those with dry or mature skin.

An FDA report on acne products states, "Some irritation occurs when benzoyl peroxide is applied to human skin. This consists of mild burning and itching in most subjects and moderate drying and peeling in all subjects."

As one might expect, the incidence and intensity of irritation increase as one increases the concentration of benzoyl peroxide. Obviously one should opt for controlling one's acne with the lowest concentration possible.

Another thing to be aware of is that benzoyl peroxide can cause irritation and swelling around the eyes, so it should never be applied to the eye area, and special care should be taken in washing your hands to make certain that you don't inadvertently rub it into your eyes. Some women are sensitive under the nostrils and around the mouth. It's a good idea to avoid that whole area. Another thing to remember is that your neck is probably going to be more sensitive than the skin on your face.

Benzoyl peroxide is a bleach and it will discolor just about any colored fabric, so if you care about your linens, use white towels and washcloths when removing it. Obviously, if it is going to touch clothing, the same thing will happen.

Caution   The FDA has the following warning to be used in products containing benzoyl peroxide. I'm quoting it because so many women don't take the time to read labels.

> Do not use this medication if you have very sensitive skin or if you are sensitive to benzoyl peroxide. This product may cause irritation, characterized by redness, burning, itching, peeling, or possible swelling. More frequent use or higher concentrations may aggravate such irritation. Mild irritation may be reduced by using the product less frequently or in a lower concentration. If irritation becomes severe, discontinue use; if irritation still continues, consult a doctor. Keep away from eyes, lips, mouth and sensitive areas of the neck. This product may bleach hair or dyed fabric.

Salicylic Acid

Salicylic acid has a long history in the treatment of acne and is often used alone or in combination with sulfur or resorcinol. However, as with other ingredients, no one is quite sure why or how it works. It is assumed that the effect of salicylic acid is as an anti-inflammatory as well as a keratolytic agent. In a twelve-week study, good or excellent results in terms of total lesions were gained by 40 percent of the patients using 2 percent salicylic acid. Salicylic acid seemed to have a very good effect on inflamed lesions such as papules and pustules.

Salicylic acid is allowed in concentrations of 0.5 to 2 percent.

Sulfur

Sulfur is one of the oldest of the modern drugs and has a long, well-documented history. Nonetheless, how it works against acne is not really known. It is assumed that it works by fighting bacteria while exfoliating the skin. Currently the highest concentration of sulfur included in over-the-counter acne products is 10 percent.

There have been a good number of double-blind studies on acne treatments that included sulfur. In one such study, one group of patients was treated with a solution of 3 percent sulfur; another group was treated with 5 percent benzoyl peroxide; one group was treated with a combination of 3 percent sulfur and 10 percent benzoyl peroxide; there was also a control group. Of the patients treated with sulfur alone, 33 percent were rated as satisfactory; with the benzoyl peroxide–sulfur combination, 54 percent were rated satisfactory; 41.7 percent of the patients using only benzoyl peroxide received a satisfactory rating; 10 percent of the control group rated satisfactory.

Many of these studies with sulfur, benzoyl peroxide, and combinations of the two were not statistically analyzed. In some studies, it was found that the combination of benzoyl peroxide and sulfur was more effective than either ingredient used alone. In other studies, there was no significant difference between the ingredients.

Sulfur can sometimes cause a mild skin sensitivity and can irritate the eyes.

Caution The FDA gives the following warning for products containing sulfur, "Do not get into eyes. If excessive skin irritation develops or increases, discontinue use and consult a doctor or pharmacist."

Benzoyl Peroxide–Sulfur Combinations

Although benzoyl peroxide and sulfur are both considered safe as single ingredients, when combined, the sulfur increases the possibility of sensitization to benzoyl peroxide. For that reason, the FDA concluded that drugs that contain both benzoyl peroxide and sulfur require monitoring by a physician. Therefore, benzoyl peroxide–sulfur combinations are not available in over-the-counter drugs and require a doctor's prescription.

If you see a dermatologist and get a prescription for this combination, it will probably be for a solution that contains 7.5 percent benzoyl peroxide and 5 percent sulfur.

Sulfur Resorcinol

Although sulfur and resorcinol are frequently used together in an effective treatment for acne, no one is really sure why it works. But several studies have been done, with good results for the combination. In one study, patients applied a cream with 8 percent sulfur and 2 percent resorcinol to one side of their faces. On the other side, they applied a placebo lotion. No other treatment besides soap and water was allowed. After eight weeks, the sulfur-resorcinol facial sides showed visual improvement in 75 percent of the cases; the placebo side improved for 46.4 percent of the patients.

In another study, 5 percent benzoyl peroxide and sulfur resorcinol were used on different sides of the face, and there was significant difference in the results.

Resorcinol by itself is not considered an effective treatment for acne, but it is believed that it enhances the activity of sulfur. The FDA allows a combination of 8 percent sulfur with 2 percent resorcinol, or 8 percent sulfur with 3 percent resorcinol monacetate.

In concentrations of 3 percent resorcinol and higher, there is some indication of local toxicity, including dermatitis, edema, itching, and peeling. There is also the possibility of systemic toxicity of a more serious nature. To guard against this, the FDA does not allow concentrations of resorcinol at more than 2 percent in over-the-counter acne medication. Resorcinol monoacetate, with a milder, but longer-lasting, effect is allowed at 3 percent.

Products containing resorcinol should not be applied to broken skin and should not be applied to large areas of the body because of the possibility of percutaneous absorption into the body. Such products should carry the following warning, "Apply to affected areas only. Do not use on broken skin or apply to large areas of the body."

If you have a dark complexion or black skin, resorcinol can sometimes cause discoloration.

Some Common Ingredients That Have Not Received Category I Status

---

There is a whole variety of ingredients that have been used over the years in acne preparations that are not considered drug ingredients. These include:

Magnesium aluminum silicate—Although this is not considered an effective treatment for acne, some products, such as oil-free foundations, include it as an ingredient because it absorbs oils.

Silica—This is another ingredient included because of its ability to absorb oil.

Camphor—Camphor is used because it feels cool; some users say that it helps relieve itching and produces a soothing effect on the skin. It does not affect the course of an acne breakout.

Menthol—This is included for many of the same reasons as camphor.

Vitamin E—Not only is there no justification in using topically applied vitamin E as an anti-acne agent, there have been some studies in which vitamin E acted as a sensitizer on the face. This seems to be particularly possible when vitamin E is used along with an acne product that has a peeling effect.

Zinc salts—Zinc over the years has been used as an astringent, a protective, and as an antiseptic, but the drug panel concludes that zinc salts (zinc oxide, zinc stearate, and zinc sulfide) have no established effectiveness in the treatment of acne.

Borates (sodium borate and boric acid)—Sodium borate may act as an abrasive in the removal of superficial acne eruptions, but, according to the FDA advisory panel, "it probably does not effectively remove the primary lesions of acne" because they are deeply rooted in the follicles.

The panel received insufficient controlled clinical evidence to support the effectiveness of boric acid and sodium borate in the treatment of acne.

Black Skin and Acne

Because of the problems connected with pigmentary changes, black skin presents special difficulties when it comes to choices of treatment.

Benzoyl peroxide, for instance, can darken skin. Retin-A can lighten it. Just the act of peeling, which is the result of using most acne products, can alter pigmentation. Some of this is temporary, but not all, and not always.

The best thing a black woman can do is to err on the side of caution when it comes to acne prevention. If you have oily skin or a tendency toward acne, be diligent in searching out and buying only noncomedegenic cosmetics. Don't let small acne flare-ups get out of control. Don't pick at your acne or do anything that might cause scarring or irritate the skin.

Several dermatologists I spoke to also advised being particularly gentle about cleansing techniques. Gentle seems to be the operative word throughout, and if you have acne, stay away from abrasives and rough cleansers.

If you do have an acne flare-up and want to use a benzoyl peroxide product, start slowly in terms of concentration and time. I spoke to a dermatologist who is knowledgeable about black skin, and it was suggested that black women start with a 2.5 benzoyl peroxide solution. The only problem with this is that I searched high and low for a product in the 2.5 range and found few stores that stocked it. You can, of course, dilute any product. Ask your pharmacist how to do this.

When you start with benzoyl peroxide, use it for only a very limited period of time, under thirty minutes. Then rinse it off. Try that for at least a week to check out the results.

If you have even a mild case of acne and feel that the threat of a pigmentation change is particularly disturbing to you, it might be a good idea to consult immediately with a dermatologist who is sensitive and well informed about black skin. If you have anything more severe than mild acne, if it is at all possible, consult an appropriate dermatologist. If you phone a dermatologist to make an appointment, don't be nervous about asking questions. Voice your concern and don't be intimidated about seeming to be overly concerned with your appearance. It's *your* face and *your* skin. Make certain that any doctor you are going to see doesn't take your concerns about pigmentation as being pure vanity and not worthy of caution and appropriate care.

When You Need a Dermatologist

Not all acne responds to self-diagnosis and treatment. Many times, particularly in adult-onset acne, you will require expert help. I cannot begin to stress enough the distinctions between different kinds of expert help. Here are some of the things you don't want to do if you have acne flare-ups.

· Don't have a facial.
· Don't visit the cosmetics counter and buy various cosmetic cleansing preparations (the efficacy of these are not to be mistaken with that of over-the-counter acne drug medications).
· Don't pick, scrub, or clean your skin.
· Don't borrow a friend's prescription medicine and self-medicate.

   Here's what you do want to do:

· Do visit a dermatologist.
· Do make certain before your visit that the doctor is someone whose philosophy of acne care is current and effective.

Some Things a Dermatologist May Do for Acne

A dermatologist may decide to prescribe a more concentrated benzoyl peroxide. Not only does this require a prescription, but the administration of it should be monitored by a physician.

   The dermatologist may prescribe retinoic acid (vitamin A acid). This is the substance that has been getting so much press as an anti-aging drug.

It was used on acne long before anyone tried it on wrinkles, and it is extremely effective. Treatment with it also requires a doctor's prescription and supervision.

The dermatologist may want to prescribe a topical antibiotic or other ointments that require monitoring and supervision.

If large cysts or severe lesions are involved, the doctor may feel that acne surgery is necessary. This procedure requires a doctor who is a skilled expert. Not all doctors perform such surgery. It definitely should not be done by yourself or by a beauty specialist who is experienced in giving facials.

The dermatologist may feel that systemic drugs are essential. In severe cases, the dermatologist, for example, may feel it is necessary to prescribe an oral antibiotic.

Until recently, dermatologists were prescribing Accutane, known generically as isotretinoin. Accutane, the only drug that seemed to work for severe cystic acne, was once believed to be a "miracle" acne drug, but then in May 1988, the FDA asked Hoffmann-La Roche, the drug's manufacturer, to take strong new measures to prevent its use by pregnant women. The reason was that at least a dozen lawsuits were beginning to be filed against Hoffmann-La Roche linking Accutane to birth defects in children born to mothers who were taking the drug. The total extent of the number of children who suffered severe birth defects because of exposure to the drug is not known, but it has been estimated as high as 25 percent. Right now the FDA has received reports of sixty-two documented cases of Accutane-linked birth defects, but there is good reason to believe that many more cases have gone unreported to date. There are also numerous other lawsuits in the works claiming other injuries of a less serious nature from the drug.

In most cases, those who are claiming injuries from the drug feel that they were not sufficiently warned of the potential dangers inherent in the drug. The manufacturer claims that dermatologists and users should have been aware of the dangers because the literature circulated was very clear in its warnings to pregnant women and women of childbearing age, who were told to practice stringent contraception while on the drug.

The current conflict revolves not only around the lawsuits, but over whether the drug should be removed altogether from the market. However, there are some people who feel that the drug's potential benefits are such that Hoffmann-La Roche should be allowed to continue to market it with careful warnings and controlled usage. Hoffmann-La Roche has suggested proposals, including physician education and limiting the drug's use only to patients with a disfiguring form of acne. *The New York Times* reports that Europe has more stringent regulations on the drug's use and that women in Britain using the drug must stipulate that they will avoid becoming pregnant while using it and agree to an immediate abortion if they do become pregnant.

Even before the Accutane-related problems surfaced, many physicians believed that the average case of acne is best controlled with topical medication; they reserve the systemic treatments for severe cases.

16

Being a Knowledgeable
Skin Care Consumer

Your Skin Care Notebook—Taking Yourself and Your Skin Seriously

I always give women this advice: Keep track of what you buy, and keep track of what you use. The best way to do this is to keep all the information in one place. To do this, you will need a large sturdy loose-leaf notebook, one that will hold up for years.

Date the first page, and at the very top, write in your age and your skin type now. Jot down how you evaluated your skin type. Did you do it by yourself? Was it done by a department store salesperson, or by a computer?

Since skin type changes, it should be reevaluated regularly. Leave room on the first few pages so you can write in your skin type at six-month intervals.

Then take a little bit of time, and record your skin care history, including a list of products that you felt improved the way you looked. List the moisturizers that have worked for you, and the ones you have discarded. If you ever had an allergic reaction to a product, write it down. If anything gave you pimples, write it down.

Then, whenever you buy a new skin care product, enter it into the notebook. Give it a page of its own, and write down the following information: name of product, type (mask, cleanser, etc.), date purchased, price, manufacturer, and anything that you think might be relevant. Cut out the ingredient label from the box and staple or clip it into the notebook along with any directions or promotional literature you received with the product. Take a look at your skin in the mirror and make a note about how it looks. Are there dry spots, pimples, clogged pores, etc.? If you have comedones, count them. Make a record of what you see on your facial skin. Then write down why you bought the product and your mood when you purchased it. Were you happy? Were you upset about something in your life? Did you feel that you experienced hardsell sales techniques?

After you have had the product about six weeks, take a look at your skin. How does it look? Are there any new problem areas? Are the old ones still there? Write down whether your skin looks better or worse and count any comedones or pimples, making note of which are new and which are old. Did the product make your skin itch or burn? Did it make your eyes itch or burn?

Note whether you are using the product regularly or if you have stopped using it and why. And most important, write down whether the product fulfilled its expectations, and whether you think the cost was worth the results.

If the product is a *moisturizer,* note the following: Did it make makeup application easier or more difficult? How did it make your skin look without makeup? Is the product quickly absorbed or does it just sit on your face feeling sticky and gooey? Do you like the texture and consistency? How long after application does the skin still feel moist?

If the product is a *cleansing mask,* note the following: After using, do your pores look smaller? How long does this effect last? Were you satisfied with the results? Does the skin look and feel tighter? Did the product irritate your skin?

If the product is a *scrub,* note the following: Did it irritate your skin? Did you experience any burning or itching after you used it? Were you satisfied or dissatisfied with the results?

If the product is an *anti-aging* cream, note the following: How long did the product last? Did anything about the product particularly please or displease you? Did you feel that it in any way gave a more youthful appearance, or less wrinkled skin? Do you think the results justified the price?

If the product is a *toner,* note the following: Did it burn or tingle or in any way indicate that it was irritating your skin? Did it make your pores appear smaller, even temporarily? How long did that effect last? Did it remove oils, grease, and dirt as it was supposed to?

If the product was an *eye cream* or an *eye gel,* note the following: Did it improve the appearance of the skin around your eyes? Did you experience any burning or itching or any other kind of reaction? Did the product fulfill the promise of the promotional literature? If it promised to reduce puffiness, do you feel that it did the job? Were the creams easy to apply or did you have to pull at your skin? Can the product be worn under eye makeup, or is it too greasy?

If the product is a *cleanser,* note the following: Does it do the job? Does it remove makeup and surface dirt and oils? Does it leave a film on the face? Does it leave the skin feeling tight and dry, indicating, perhaps, that the pH is too alkaline for your skin? Does it leave your skin soft and smooth? Do you like the smell?

Whenever you replace the same product, make a note of it in your notebook. Compare the ingredient labels of the old and the new product. Are they the same? If there are any changes in the ingredients, cut out the new label, date it and clip it in with the old.

This notebook can be invaluable if you have any form of irritation or breakout because it can often help you pinpoint offending ingredients. It's also a useful way of helping you understand how you spend your skin care dollars and whether you are getting your money's worth. It wipes away the confusion that we all sometimes feel after trying a new product because it helps you keep track of your wrinkles and blemishes and the way in which products affect them.

Final Advice for Shoppers: Twelve Things to Remember at the Cosmetics Counter

Whether they are wearing lab coats, frilly silk blouses, or Dior suits, those attractive men and women behind the cosmetics counter have been trained to *sell.* There is every possibility that they have attended seminars in selling, read company-inspired literature on selling, and/or trained with a more experienced person. Their primary goal is to convince you to buy their products.

The companies have done other things as well. They have spent millions on advertising, packaging, and promotion to create an attitude and an image. At least half of what you will be told will probably be questionable. Keep this in mind. Unless you, the consumer, also develop an attitude, you are simply too vulnerable.

When you shop, you need to have a certain amount of defensiveness in your attitude. You can't be intimidated, and you have to be assertive about your needs. The attitude of the skin care salesperson varies from store to store, obviously. In my experience, he or she is most likely to get annoyed in large, big-city cosmetics departments and be most helpful in smaller outlets. Whatever the attitude of the salesperson, remember, it's your money, and you have the right to ask questions before you spend a lot of dollars on a couple of ounces of face cream.

At the Skin Care Counter

1. Read the ingredients label.

This is not so easy to do. The packaging is not out in the open, and there is a great deal of resistance on the part of some companies to the notion of consumers reading the ingredients label. You have the right to look at the ingredients label to see whether the ingredients reflect the promotion and the literature. When you look at the label, remember that the ingredients are listed in descending order of concentration. Look to make certain the product is designed for your skin type. Is there anything listed to which you are sensitive? Are the ingredients important for your skin type?

2. At the beginning, buy small.

If it is the first time you are buying the product, don't be sold on the premise that buying larger sizes will save money. You might take the product home and stop using it. If the product works, and you are happy with the results, you can always buy the larger size when you run out.

3. Don't be intimidated by overly aggressive or overly solicitous skin care salespeople.

Cosmetics salespeople tend to approach a consumer the moment she stops to browse. Consequently, some women never get past the counter nearest the door. If you want to look at all the various skin care counters before deciding what, if anything, you want to buy, take the time to do so.

4. Don't be afraid to ask questions, and don't be embarrassed about walking away without buying after you have the answers.

Remember that you have the right to take your time before making skin care purchases, so ask as many questions as you like. The salesperson is supposed to be trained to answer your questions.

5. Buy only what you can afford.

There are lots of good products in all price ranges. Remember that most dermatologists say that good old inexpensive petrolatum is still the best moisturizer, so don't buy that $60 moisturizer unless you can afford it.

6. Don't be snowed by the white coats or the complicated language.

There are very few Ph.D.s out selling cosmetics, white coats notwithstanding. Keep that in mind when your salesperson begins to roll off pseudoscientific terminology.

7. Don't believe in miracles.

Some companies have toned down the claims on their promotional literature. Other companies still use some of the same words as before, and many of the salespeople still speak of miraculous results.

8. Don't buy a skin care product just to get the free gift.

Some companies regularly offer a free gift with a purchase. Many of these are truly nice gifts. However, many women end up buying a product they don't want just to get a mini-kit or a travel kit that they are never going to use. Unless you truly want the product, don't be induced into buying it because of the free gift.

9. Don't become a skin care junkie.

Trying product line after product line can be disastrous for your skin as well as for your pocketbook.

10. Don't rush to buy skin care products after a makeover or a facial.

Wait until you get home and think about which products you really want to buy. Then go back and buy them once you are sure that none of them have irritated your skin, that you really want and need them, that you really can afford them, and that you really will use them. It's too easy to get overwhelmed after a facial. Some women feel guilty about the operator; others just throw caution to the wind and buy whatever strikes their fancy at the moment; and still others are talked into buying products they don't want. Wait. You can always go back to the store in a few days.

11. Watch out for a tendency to buy skin care extras that will never be used or that will run up your bill.

There is a whole variety of expensive products and extras sold that the typical consumer doesn't need. If you don't need it, don't buy it.

12. When buying a new skin care product, remember to get instructions.

Instructions are frequently omitted on skin care products, both on the outside and the inside packaging. Before purchasing a product, you should ask two questions:

How many times a day do I use this product?

This is extremely important. Some products for oily skin, for example, are much too drying to be used indiscriminately. Someplace, somewhere, someone in the company has tested the product and knows exactly how often it should be used. Make certain you get this information. If the salesperson doesn't know, ask her to call the company's consumer representative and find out.

How much of this product do I use?

Often only a small amount is required, but many women use more and waste money. Ask. Someone has the answer to this question as well.

Summing It All Up

· Use as few products as possible.

Basic skin care is not that complicated, and chances are that trying to make it more complicated than it really is, is only going to benefit the manufacturers' wallets. Remember that it isn't good for your skin to get too much handling. Complicated rituals are often not only time-consuming and expensive. Some are potentially harmful and can lead to dermatological problems.

Common sense is the key. Limit the number and types of creams and lotions to those that are absolutely essential.

· Handle your skin as little as possible.

Unnecessary touching, manipulating, squeezing, and massaging can irritate and inflame your skin. It can give you pimples and even induce certain forms of acne. Keep all removals and applications of makeup and skin care products as simple as possible and avoid prolonged scrubbing with skin care products.

· If your skin becomes irritated by a specific skin care program or line of cosmetics, do not rush right out to find something new.

If you find that you develop sensitivity to a particular product or line of products, wait at least two weeks, preferably longer, before you start looking for something new. Sensitive skin is sensitive skin. Under ordinary circumstances it cannot just be blamed on a particular product. You have to let your skin "calm down" before you try anything else. If these irritations are a frequent occurrence, you should visit a dermatologist and evaluate your skin care regimen to see whether or not you can design a program that will be less irritating.

· If your skin becomes irritated or breaks out or if small white bumps start to appear under your skin, stop using all skin care and makeup products until you figure out what's causing the problem.

An allergic dermatitis usually doesn't erupt the first time you use a product. It can happen even when it's something that you've been using for years. Also, it can take several weeks for a pimple or comedones to develop. Cosmetic acne typically doesn't occur for four to six weeks after one begins applying the particular comedegenic ingredients. If the breakout is not mild or it doesn't clear up, consult a dermatologist immediately—not a cosmetics salesperson.

· If you have a reaction to a particular product or product line, return the products with the sales slip to the cosmetics department where they were bought. Most companies will give you credit. Do not immediately buy a new group of products. For example, if you got cosmetic acne from a moisturizer, don't let yourself be convinced that you need the company's oily skin products. They may be right for you, or they may not. But your skin needs several weeks to calm down. And you may need to consult a dermatologist to examine the ingredients you used on your skin in order to determine what you should or should not use.

· Keep in mind that many products have a predetermined shelf life.

Some skin care products are filled with oils, which can eventually become rancid even though there are preservatives in the formula. If you want to extend the life of your expensive creams, lotions, and other potions, keep them refrigerated.

· Do not plaster your skin with a plethora of skin care products, believing that one or a combination of them will miraculously reduce your wrinkles, control your acne, or alter your destiny.

At this time, according to the FDA, the only cosmetic product that can make a legitimate anti-aging claim is a sunscreen with an approved sunscreen ingredient and an SPF number.

Cosmetic skin care products are not drugs and they are not magical potions. If you have real skin problems, see a real dermatologist. I think every skin care consumer should understand that the chances are very slim that a skin care line will be effective in dealing with medical or physiological problems such as acne or aging.

· Remember: the dermatologist is the expert.

The most vital information I can give you is to stress how important a function skin plays not only in how we look, but in how we feel. Many women who have a skin problem, of any kind, have a tendency to run to the "beauty expert" at the cosmetics counter or the facial salon before they run to the dermatologist. This is generally unwise, and while I realize the high cost of medical care, in the long run it can often save you money to start out by doing the prudent thing. Any skin problem that does not go away within a reasonable period of time or recurs requires an expert's evaluation and diagnosis.

INDEX

About the Author

Elaine Brumberg is a cosmetics consumer advocate and beauty consultant. Hailed as the Ralph Nader of the cosmetics industry, she has conducted seminars for major department stores, lectured at national conventions, served as a consultant to well-known cosmetic surgeons, and appeared frequently on radio and television talk shows, including "Donahue," "Good Morning America," and "CNN News Night." She has her own consulting firm, which advises women on how to buy and properly apply cosmetics, how to cope with aging, and how to put their best face forward through clothing, makeup, and body language. She is the mother of four adult children and is a grandmother. She and her husband live in the Philadelphia area.

I would like to know more about your beauty problems, from your head to your toes. If you have questions concerning cosmetic surgery, hair, skin, or makeup color and/or application or would like to share your "trade secret" facials or beauty tips, send all questions and/or tips to

Elaine Brumberg
P.O. Box 301
Jenkintown, PA 19046